Core Psychopharmacology

Pádraig Wright MB MRCPsych MD
Honorary Senior Lecturer
Institute of Psychiatry
London

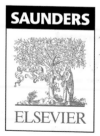

SAUNDERS

ELSEVIER

Edinburgh London New York Oxford Philadelphia St Louis Sydney Toronto 2006

SAUNDERS

ELSEVIER

An imprint of Elsevier Limited

First published 2006

ISBN 10: 0702028126
ISBN 13: 9780702028120

British Library Cataloguing in Publication Data
A catalogue record for this book is available from the British Library

Library of Congress Cataloging in Publication Data
A catalog record for this book is available from the Library of Congress

Notice

Knowledge and best practice in this field are constantly changing. As new research and experience broaden our knowledge, changes in practice, treatment and drug therapy may become necessary or appropriate. Readers are advised to check the most current information provided (i) on procedures featured or (ii) by the manufacturer of each product to be administered, to verify the recommended dose or formula, the method and duration of administration, and contraindications. It is the responsibility of the practitioner, relying on their own experience and knowledge of the patient, to make diagnoses, to determine dosages and the best treatment for each individual patient, and to take all appropriate safety precautions. To the fullest extent of the law, neither the publisher nor the author assumes any liability for any injury and/or damage to persons or property arising out or related to any use of the material contained in this book.

The Publisher

Printed in China

Preface

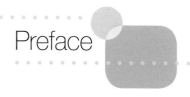

'Doctors are men who prescribe medicines of which they know little, to cure diseases of which they know less, in humans beings of whom they know nothing.'

Voltaire (1694–1778)

The science of psychopharmacology is progressing rapidly and the number and variety of psychotropic drugs with which a psychiatrist must be familiar is increasing all the time. These drugs are a vital component of the treatment of many patients suffering from psychiatric illness. My hope is that this book may help psychiatrists, general practitioners and others become clinicians '... who prescribe psychotropic medicines of which they know quite a lot ...'.

This textbook of psychopharmacology is written by a clinical psychopharmacologist working in the pharmaceutical industry who is also a practising psychiatrist. My intention in writing it was to provide a single volume reference that is both an account of contemporary psychopharmacology and a summary of information from important sources that a clinician would normally have to interrogate separately. Such sources include the psychiatric research literature, the advice of national and international statutory, scientific and professional organisations, the Summary of Product Characteristics for individual drugs and the British National Formulary.

Core Psychopharmacology is divided into two parts. Part I provides an overview of Basic Psychopharmacology. Part II provides a detailed account of Clinical Psychopharmacology and discusses every class of psychotropic drug, and many of the individual psychotropic drugs, with which clinicians practising in the United Kingdom and Ireland must be familiar. The advice of organisations including the National Institute for Clinical Excellence, the Committee on Safety of Medicines and The Royal College of Psychiatrists is also incorporated into Part II.

Core Psychopharmacology is intended primarily as a postgraduate textbook for candidates studying for the Part I and Part II membership examinations of the Royal College of Psychiatrists and other similar examinations. I believe it will also be of value to general practitioners – who prescribe the great bulk of psychotropic drugs – and to neurologists, clinical psychologists and psychiatric nurses.

Pádraig Wright
London, 2006

Contents

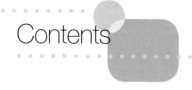

Contents

Contents

Part I

Basic Psycopharmacology

1

Introduction to basic psychopharmacology

The syllabus for the Part I and Part II membership examinations of the Royal College of Psychiatrists requires a trainee psychiatrist to have:

- an awareness of the history and development of psychotropic drugs
- a working knowledge of neurotransmission
- a working knowledge of the pharmacokinetics and pharmacodynamics of psychotropic drugs and
- an awareness of psychotropic drug development and of regulatory issues.

Part I of this book consists of four chapters that address each of these topics in turn. However, knowledge of these topics is not only essential for candidates intending to take the Part I and Part II membership examinations. It is also essential to the practice of psychiatry. It is not possible to prescribe psychotropic drugs rationally without a good understanding of neurotransmission and of their pharmacokinetics and pharmacodynamics. Nor is it possible to adequately explain the benefits and risks of psychotropic drugs to patients without this knowledge. And given that psychotropic drugs are one of the principal weapons in a psychiatrist's therapeutic armamentarium it seems reasonable to expect that all psychiatrists have an awareness of their history and of how such drugs are invented, developed, licensed and monitored.

2

A history of psychopharmacology

Introduction

Elephants and pigs have long been observed to enjoy the effects of alcohol obtained by eating fallen mangoes or apples that are fermenting. It seems likely that our ancestors observed and copied the behaviour of such animals and then, being human, developed methods by which a continuous supply of alcohol could be ensured. In any case they had learned how to produce alcohol at least 9000 years ago. One assumes that the survival value of such learning was then, as now, the desire for temporary escape from the human condition. But it is inevitable that such escape was provided by naturally occurring psychotropic substances obtained from plants and including tobacco, cannabis, opium and coffee during the millennia that constituted what may be called the pre-alcoholic era. Recreational psychopharmacology is therefore a very old science.

Therapeutic as distinct from recreational psychopharmacology is a relatively young science. It was founded as the 19th century drew to a close and continues to flourish today. This chapter provides an account of the early history of psychopharmacology, the physical treatments employed before the contemporary era of psychopharmacology and contemporary psychopharmacology itself. It concludes with a brief commentary on the future of psychopharmacology.

Early psychopharmacology

Plants were used for recreational, ceremonial and medicinal purposes in prehistoric times. The earliest and best known written records of such use include:

- the code of 282 laws formulated by Hammurabi (c. 1810–1750 BC), the sixth king of Babylon, and inscribed on a stone stela found at Susa in 1901
- the Smith (c. 1600 BC) and Ebers (c. 1500 BC) papyri from Thebes, the latter of which is generally regarded as the first medical textbook
- the cuneiform inscribed clay tablets from the library of Assurbanipal (c. 668–627 BC) from Nineveh and
- the writings of Dioscorides (c. 40–90 AD), the Greek surgeon to the Roman emperor Nero, whose *Materia Medica* produced in 65 AD included a list of 500 medicinal plants and remained in circulation for 1600 years.

All of the above records refer to medical practice within the context of religious ritual and indeed physician and priest were often one and the same. Furthermore, these records did not differentiate between illnesses affecting the body and those affecting the mind. Hippocrates (c. 460–377 BC) distinguished between medicine and religion and, in addition to encouraging his patients to eat healthily and exercise regularly, also promoted the judicial use of drugs. If we now leap from antiquity to the 16th century AD – ignoring the contributions of civilisations such as those of ancient China and India (including *Rauwolfia* – see below) and of individuals such as Galen (130–200 AD) and Avicienna (980–1037 AD) as we do – we reach the time of Paracelsus. It is to him we must turn for both the first recognition of mental illness as a disease of the mind and for the first steps in psychopharmacology.

Theophrastus Phillippus Aureolus Bombastus von Hohenheimor (1493–1541), better known as Paracelsus, has been called the grand-father of pharmacology. He believed that nature had provided a specific treatment for every illness ('… *there is always some remedy, a herb against one, a stone against another, a mineral against one, a poison against another, a metal against one, something else against another…*') and thus that drugs should be administered alone rather than in combination. But perhaps his best known adage is that it is the dosage in which a substance is administered that determines whether it is a drug or a poison. The drugs administered by Paracelsus were made in his laboratory and were herbs (many of which had anticholinergic activity), minerals or heavy metals. They included opium, belladonna, hyoscine, caffeine, iron, copper, sulphur, camphor, arsenic, lead and mercury. He conducted a primitive clinical trial of mercury in the treatment of epilepsy and found it to be effective.

Physical treatments before psychopharmacology

The history of the physical treatments employed in the battle against mental illness in the decades preceding the introduction of effective psychotropic drugs has been well-documented. The key treatments and their discoverers are as follows:

- Malaria therapy for psychosis was proposed by the Austrian Julius Werner von Jauregg (1857–1940) in 1887. This treatment was effective in alleviating the relatively high proportion of psychoses that was caused by general paralysis of the insane in von Jauregg's day, because high fever is lethal to *Treponema pallidum*. Malaria therapy was ineffective against non-syphilitic psychoses.

- Insulin coma therapy for schizophrenia was introduced by the German Manfred Joshua Sakel (1900–1957) in 1934. This very hazardous treatment became commonplace in psychiatric hospitals during the 1940s and 1950s but it was ultimately proven to be ineffective in alleviating schizophrenia.

- Convulsive therapy for schizophrenia was introduced by the Hungarian Ladislas Joseph von Meduna (1896–1964) in 1934, based on the observation that patients rarely suffered from both epilepsy and schizophrenia. Convulsive therapy was effective for some patients but the camphor (and later metrazol) used by von Meduna did not cause immediate unconsciousness and induced seizures of such intensity as to cause vertebral fracture.

- Frontal leucotomy for schizophrenia and depression was developed by the Portuguese Egas Moniz (1874–1955) in 1935. Many thousands of patients received this treatment before its adverse effects were realised. Today, approximately 20 surgical procedures (subcaudate tractotomy, anterior cingulotomy, anterior capsulotomy and limbic leucotomy) are performed annually in the UK in patients with treatment-resistant disorders, predominantly depression, bipolar disorder, obsessive compulsive disorder and anxiety.

- Electroconvulsive therapy for schizophrenia was developed by the Italians Ugo Cerletti (1877–1963) and Lucio Bini (1908–1964) in 1938. This treatment remains in use, albeit much modified and almost exclusively for the treatment of depression, to this day.

Contemporary psychopharmacology

In the beginning

A number of sedating drugs became available during the second half of the 19th century. The first of these, paraldehyde was invented in 1828 by the German chemist Hermann von Fehling (1812–1885) and became available through the Bayer company in 1882. Over 120 years later it is still occasionally used in the treatment of status epilepticus and severe agitation.

Chloral hydrate was invented by the German chemist Justus Baron von Liebig (1803–1873) (who also developed the Oxo cube, marketing it through his own company, Lemco) in 1832. Chloral hydrate became available through the Bayer company in 1888 and remains in use today.

Potassium bromide was first used by the Englishman Sir Charles Locock (1799–1875) in 1857 for treating epilepsy and reducing libido. It and other bromides (including lithium bromide – see below) were widely used towards the end of the 19th and during the early decades of the 20th centuries, both for the treatment of epilepsy and as general sedatives. They are no longer used today.

Barbituric acid was invented in 1864 by the German chemist Johann Friedrich Wilhelm Adolf von Bayer (1835–1917). Diethyl barbiturate was invented by the Germans Emil Fischer (1852–1919) and Joseph von Mering (1849–1908) in 1902 and became available as a hypnotic through the Bayer and Schering companies in 1904 under the brand names Veronal (said to be chosen in tribute to the peaceful atmosphere of the Italian city of Verona) and Medinal respectively. This drug and its successors such as phenobarbital, introduced in 1912 as Luminal by Bayer, were widely used in psychiatric hospitals until the 1970s to induce sleep extending over several days in patients with schizophrenia. They were also widely used to treat insomnia and anxiety. However, this led to barbiturate dependency which became widespread during the first half of the 20th century. Barbiturates are used to a limited extent today in the treatment of epilepsy and intractable insomnia and in anaesthesia.

Amfetamines were invented in 1887 by the German chemist L Edeleano. Dexamfetamine and methamfetamine were introduced for the treatment of narcolepsy and attention deficit hyperactivity disorder in 1937 as Dexidrine by the Smith, Kline and French company and Methedrine by Burroughs Wellcome. They were widely misused almost immediately because of their stimulant effect and this also led to their being distributed to US, British, German and Japanese soldiers during World War II. Amfetamine dependency became widespread from the 1950s onwards and remains a significant problem. Amfetamines remain in use for the treatment of narcolepsy and attention deficit hyperactivity disorder.

Phenytoin was invented in 1908 by the German chemist Heinrich Blitz. Its antiepileptic properties were not discovered until 1937 and it was made available by the Parke Davis company in 1938. It continues to be used widely as a first-line treatment for generalised epilepsy with tonic clonic seizures.

The modern era – the 1950s

The modern era of psychopharmacology began in the middle of the 20th century and has enjoyed two golden decades to date. The first of these, the 1950s approximately, saw the discovery and subsequent introduction of the nine drugs or classes of drugs which will now be described and of which all but reserpine remain in use today.

Disulfiram

Disulfiram was invented in 1948 as an anthelmintic by the Danish chemists Erik Jacobsen and Jens Hald working at the Medicinalco company. They subsequently proposed its use in alcohol dependency when, having taken disulfiram to treat worms with which they had become infested during their research, they drank alcohol and became violently ill. Disulfiram first saw clinical use in the department of Jean Delay at Hôpital Sainte-Anne, Paris, in 1949 (see chlorpromazine below).

Lithium

Lithium bromide was in use at the end of the 19th century as a general sedative but it was the Australian psychiatrist, John Frederick Joseph Cade (1912–1980), who discovered lithium's antimanic effect. Cade was investigating the hypothesis that mania was caused by excess urea by injecting lithium urate, the most soluble urate salt available, into guinea pigs. He found that it caused not hyperactivity as expected but marked sedation and subsequently investigated its effects in manic patients. Cade's 1949 publication received little attention but it led Mogens Schou (1918 to present), a Danish psychiatrist, to undertake a series of clinical trials of lithium during the 1950s. These and subsequent studies ultimately led to lithium becoming available through the Ciba-Geigy company and to its universal use as a prophylactic agent in bipolar illness.

Chlorpromazine

Chlorpromazine was invented by the French chemist Paul Charpentier of the Rhône-Poulenc company in 1950 and was subsequently used by

Henri Marie Laborit (1914–1995), a French naval surgeon, to induce hypothermia during anaesthesia. It was first used to treat psychosis by Jean Delay (1907–1987) and Pierre Deniker (1917–1998) at Hôpital Sainte-Anne, Paris, in 1952. Delay and Deniker reported that chlorpromazine not only calmed patients as distinct from sedating them but also alleviated their psychotic symptoms, Delay coining the term 'neuroleptic' to describe the drug's effects. Jean Thuillier, Delay's assistant, described the effect of chlorpromazine graphically when he wrote '…the most evident sign of this extraordinary therapeutic result could be appreciated even from the outside of the building of the men's clinic – there was silence' (1999).

Reserpine

The *Rauwolfia* plant had been used to treat mental illness in India for hundreds of years and in 1952 Hugo Bein of the Ciba company isolated reserpine, its active ingredient. This was prescribed more frequently than chlorpromazine during the early 1950s but its use soon decreased because it caused akathisia in many patients treated with it and was thought – probably erroneously – to cause depression.

Monoamine oxidase inhibitors

The antidepressant effects of isoniazid, a known monoamine oxidase inhibitor (MAOI), had been noted by clinicians using it to treat patients with tuberculosis in the early 1950s. Iproniazid, another MAOI, was invented in 1957 by the Hoffman-LaRoche company as an anti-tuberculous agent. It was found to be ineffective but it was subsequently tested as an antidepressant, found to be effective and widely prescribed. It was quickly withdrawn from use because of hepato-toxicity but it paved the way for subsequent MAOIs such as phenelzine and tranylcypromine.

Imipramine

This was invented by the Geigy company as a variant on the chlorpromazine molecule. Roland Kuhn, a Swiss psychiatrist, found that it excessively stimulated patients with schizophrenia. He therefore administered it to patients with severe depression in 1955 and found it to be effective. Imipramine became the first tricyclic antidepressant drug.

Meprobamate

This was invented in the 1940s by Frank Berger, a Czechoslovak bacteriologist working with the Carter Wallace company. Meprobamate was marketed in 1954 as Miltown and hailed as the first 'tranquilliser', a word coined to describe its ability to calm patients without sedating them.

Haloperidol

The Belgian physician and chemist, Paul Janssen (1926–2003), of the eponymous pharmaceutical company, invented haloperidol in 1958. He was searching for a treatment for amfetamine toxicity, commonly experienced by professional cyclists, and had noticed the similarities between their symptoms and those of patients with schizophrenia. Haloperidol soon displaced chlorpromazine as the most frequently prescribed antipsychotic drug.

Benzodiazepines

Chlordiazepoxide, the first bendodiazepine, was invented in 1955 by the Austrian, Leo H Sternbach (1908 to present) of Hoffman-LaRoche, and introduced in 1960 under the brand name Librium. It was followed by diazepam under the brand name Valium in 1965. The benzodiazepines were hailed as safe successors to the addictive barbiturates, Valium became the most widely prescribed drug of the 1970s and the Rolling Stones immortalised it in the song 'Mother's Little Helper'. However, benzodiazepine dependency was soon recognised and was formally described by Petursson and Lader in 1981. Over 40 benzodiazepine drugs are available worldwide today and, while their use has declined, they retain an important place in psychiatry in the treatment of severe anxiety, panic disorder and insomnia and in detoxification from alcohol.

I have presented the drugs listed above in chronological order by their dates of invention. This suggests a steady progression in neuroscience, pharmaceutical development and clinical psychiatry. This is far from the truth. Progress was often piecemeal and by chance and it must be appreciated that it depended upon close interaction between the inventors of the drugs (laboratory chemists working with predominantly German chemical or pharmaceutical companies), the psychiatrists who initially prescribed and studied them and their patients who volunteered (and, in the early years, who did not volunteer) to participate in clinical research.

The modern era – the 1980s

The second golden decade of psychopharmacology, the 1980s approximately, was marked by the introduction of psychotropic drugs with either relatively selective and/or relatively novel mechanisms of action. Six different groups of drugs warrant description.

Atypical antipsychotic drugs

Clozapine, the archetypal atypical antipsychotic drug (the term 'atypical' refers to the fact that it does not cause catalepsy in laboratory animals and has a lower risk for extrapyramidal and other adverse effects in patients when compared with 'typical' antipsychotic drugs such as haloperidol), was invented in 1958 by Fritz Hunziker, J Schmutz and E Eichenberger of the Swiss company, Wander AG. It was not long in clinical use before it became evident that it was associated with a significant risk of agranulocytosis and it was therefore withdrawn from use in almost all countries. However, pressure from the psychiatric community led to a clinical study being undertaken by the Sandoz-Wander company in patients with treatment-resistant schizophrenia. Clozapine proved to be dramatically superior to chlorpromazine (Kane et al, 1988). It was subsequently reintroduced for clinical use in patients with treatment-resistant schizophrenia with the proviso of regular monitoring for blood dyscrasias. These licensing factors led to clozapine being termed a second-line atypical antipsychotic drug while its successors such as risperidone (invented in 1984 by Paul Janssen – see above) and olanzapine (invented in 1986 by Jiban Chakrabarti, David Tupper and Terrence Hotten of the Eli Lilly company) were licensed for the treatment of any patient with schizophrenia and are termed first-line atypical antipsychotic drugs (see Chapter 8).

Selective serotonin reuptake inhibitor antidepressant drugs

The first selective serotonin reuptake inhibitor (SSRI) was zimelidine, marketed by Astra in 1982 but soon withdrawn from clinical use because it very occasionally caused Guillain–Barré syndrome. Fluoxetine is therefore usually regarded as the first successful SSRI. It was invented in 1972 by Bryan Molley (1939–2004), David Wong (1936 to present) and Ray Fuller (1935–1996) of Eli Lilly. As Prozac, it became one of the most frequently prescribed, and written about, drugs of all time (see Chapter 9).

Selective noradrenaline (norepinephrine) reuptake inhibitor drugs

Atomoxetine, a selective noradrenaline reuptake inhibitor, was invented for the treatment of depression in the 1980s by scientists at Eli Lilly. It proved ineffective as an antidepressant but it was subsequently developed as the first non-stimulant drug for the treatment of attention deficit hyperactivity disorder (see Chapter 7).

Serotonin and noradrenaline (norepinephrine) reuptake inhibitor antidepressant drugs

Venlafaxine, the first serotonin and noradrenaline reuptake inhibitor (SNRI), was invented by John Yardley, Morris Husbands and Eric Muth of the Wyeth company in 1986 (see Chapter 9).

Selective phosphodiesterase type 5 inhibitor drugs

Sildenafil, the first selective phosphodiesterase type 5 inhibitor, was invented in 1989 for the treatment of hypertension and angina pectoris by Simon Campbell, David Roberts and Nick Terrett, chemists with the Pfizer company. Healthy male volunteers participating in initial clinical trials reported an increased frequency of erections. This unexpected effect led to sildenafil being developed and eventually licensed for the treatment of erectile dysfunction as Viagra in 1998 (see Chapter 13).

Anticholinesterase inhibitors and glutamate receptor antagonists

Tacrine, the first anticholinesterase inhibitor and the first drug approved for the treatment of Alzheimer's disease, was licensed in the USA in 1993. It was soon followed by donepezil, rivastigmine and galantamine, and by the glutamate receptor antagonist, memantine, in 2002 (see Chapter 16).

Drug discovery to date may be likened to collecting mushrooms. You never know precisely where you will find mushrooms but you do know with absolute certainty that you will not find any unless you are out searching for them. Thus the search for an anthelmintic led to disulfiram, for a hypothermic to chlorpromazine, for an antituberculous agent to the monoamine oxidase inhibitors and for an anti-hypertensive and antianginal agent to sildenafil. But drug discovery has been changing, rapidly and dramatically.

The future of psychopharmacology

It is said that prediction is difficult, especially about the future. However, advances in the following scientific and technical areas are already having a major influence on the discovery and development of drugs for the treatment of neuropsychiatric disorders. It seems likely that they will continue to do so, at least during the next decade or so. Potential future developments in the psychotropic drugs used to treat individual psychiatric disorders are discussed later in this book in the appropriate chapters.

Combinatorial chemistry and high-throughput screening

Combinatorial chemistry was developed in an effort to increase the rate at which new drugs are discovered and to reduce the cost of their discovery. Traditional pharmaceutical chemists synthesised, purified and tested an individual molecule. Combinatorial pharmaceutical chemists in contrast:

- synthesise vast numbers of different molecules in a single container from a known group of reactants (such libraries may include several billion molecules) and
- fix them to a polymeric support and test them for biological activity *en masse* (high-throughput screening).

Combinatorial chemistry has been made possible by advances in robotics and bioinformatics. It allows for the synthesis and testing of an almost infinite number of molecules.

Genetics

Genetics may contribute to psychotropic drug development in two very important ways.

First, if genes are found that cause specific psychiatric disorders it is possible to determine the enzyme or structural protein they code for and thus to increase our understanding of the disease. This may allow the development of a more effective and safer drug or, possibly, the development of a gene therapy through which the disease-causing gene is repaired or replaced. Gene therapy for Alzheimer's disease in which the gene for nerve growth factor (contained within a viral vector) is injected directly into the nucleus basalis of Meynert is currently being investigated in patients.

Second, pharmacogenomics may allow the development of drugs that are tailor made for the individual and therefore more effective and safer. Pharmacogenomics relies on the fact that:

- many drugs target enzymes and neuroreceptors, proteins that are coded for by genes that exhibit significant variation between individuals, and that
- while clinical studies provide reliable data on the efficacy and safety of a drug in a population of patients, it remains impossible to predict which drug will suit which individual patient with any accuracy.

Pharmacogenomics investigates the effect of genetic variation on an individual's response to drugs in the hope that genotyping patients may ultimately allow individualisation of prescribing. The only practical application of pharmacogenomics today is the case of the cytochrome P450 family of liver enzymes that are responsible for metabolising many psychotropic and other drugs. Genetic variation in the genes that code for these enzymes may significantly reduce ('slow metabolisers') or increase ('rapid metabolisers') ability to metabolise drugs such as tricyclic antidepressants and lead to adverse effects or poor treatment response.

Perhaps the most surprising outcome of the 13-year Human Genome Project that was completed in 2003 is that we have approximately 30,000 protein-coding genes rather than the 100,000 that had been predicted. For comparison, earthworms have approximately 20,000 protein-coding genes. However, proteins may be dissembled and reassembled to produce vast numbers of further proteins and pharmacogenomics has now been joined by the new science of pharmacoproteomics which has similar, if dramatically more complex, goals of increased understanding of disease and increased individualisation of drug treatment.

Pharmacoelectroencephalography

Computerised analysis of digital electrencephalography (EEG) data has led to a resurgence of interest in the effects of drugs on the EEG and the clinical interpretation of such effects. It is already possible to reliably determine the effect of a drug on sleep architecture and EEG 'fingerprints' have been determined for several classes of psychoactive drugs. It is proposed that these fingerprints may act as 'biomarkers' that allow the selection of drugs for further testing i.e. if the EEG fingerprint of a newly invented molecule is similar to that of a known antidepressant drug, the new molecule may itself be a suitable candidate for investigation as an antidepressant drug.

Neuroimaging

Structural magnetic resonance imaging and several functional neuroimaging techniques have made an increasing contribution to psychotropic drug development over the last decade.

Structural magnetic resonance imaging

It may be somewhat surprising to learn that structural neuroimaging has a role to play in psychotropic drug development. Magnetic resonance imaging (MRI) has demonstrated that patients experiencing a first episode of schizophrenia have abnormalities of grey and white matter and that these are progressive. A recent MRI study has shown that when such patients are treated with haloperidol they experience significant reductions in grey matter volume compared to peers treated with olanzapine (Lieberman et al, 2005). It is unclear whether halopridol is neurotoxic and exacerbates the schizophrenia disease process or olanzapine is neuroprotective. However, this example serves to illustrate the contribution structural MRI may make to psychotropic drug development.

Positron emission tomography

Positron emission tomography (PET) depends on the administration of biologically active molecules labelled with radioactive isotopes and their subsequent detection as positrons. It allows quantitative imaging of the effects of psychotropic drugs on metabolic processes such as regional cerebral blood flow (using water labelled with ^{15}O) and regional cerebral glucose metabolism (using deoxyglucose labelled with ^{18}F). PET also allows quantitative imaging of neuroreceptors via ligands labelled with radioactive isotopes designed to bind to specific receptors. For example, ^{11}C raclopride binds to dopamine D_2 receptors and any drug that prevents such binding is therefore confirmed as a dopamine D_2 receptor ligand.

Single photon emission tomography

Single photon emission tomography (SPET) depends on the administration of radioactive isotopes and the subsequent detection of gamma photons. It allows imaging similar to that of PET but resolution and quantification are poorer. On the other hand SPET is more readily available and less expensive than PET.

Functional magnetic resonance imaging

Functional MRI (fMRI) depends on the fact that increased neuronal activity requires metabolic energy and leads to increased regional cerebral blood flow. This alters the MR signal from nearby hydrogen nuclei (because deoxygenated haemoglobin is paramagnetic) and thus permits imaging. The importance of fMRI in evaluating the effects of psychotropic drugs on brain function is growing rapidly because it has excellent temporal and spatial resolution and does not involve the use of ionising radiation.

Magnetic resonance spectroscopy

MR spectroscopy (MRS) depends on the detection of protium [^1H] and other isotopes that possess nuclear spin such as fluorine [^{19}F], sodium [^{23}Na], phosphorus [^{31}P] and lithium [^7Li]. It allows quantification of brain neurochemistry and the production of metabolite maps of the brain. The metabolites that are most easily detected by MRS are N-acetyl aspartate which is found exclusively in neurons, creatine-1-phosphocreatine and choline. MRS is increasingly used to evaluate the effects of psychotropic drugs on brain neurochemistry.

References and further reading

Cade JFJ (1949) Lithium salts in the treatment of psychotic excitement. Medical Journal of Australia 36:349–352.

Cookson J (2004) A brief history of psychiatry. In: Core Psychiatry (Eds Wright P, Phelan M and Stern J) (2nd Edition). London, Elsevier Saunders, pp. 3–11.

Healy D (1996) The Psychopharmacologists. London, Chapman and Hall, 587 pp.

Kane J, Honigfeld G, Singer J et al (1988) Clozapine for the treatment-resistant schizophrenic. A double-blind comparison with chlorpromazine. Archives of General Psychiatry 45(9):789–796.

Lieberman JA, Tollefson GD, Charles C et al (2005) Antipsychotic drug effects on brain morphology in first-episode psychosis. Archives of General Psychiatry 62(4):361–370.

Petursson H, Lader MH (1981) Withdrawal from long term benzodiazepine treatment. British Medical Journal 283:643–645.

Porter R (Ed) (1997) Psychiatry. In: The Greatest Benefit to Mankind. London, Harper Collins, pp. 493–524.

Thuillier J (Ed) (1999) The snake pit. In: Ten Years that Changed the Face of Mental Illness. London, Martin Dunitz, pp. 19–29.

3

Neurotransmitters and neuroreceptors

Introduction

Life is neurotransmission and psychopharmacology is the science of influencing neurotransmission. Life is neurotransmission not only in the sense that vital functions essential to life depend on neurotransmission but also in the sense that conscious experience of human life depends upon it. It is dissatisfaction with this conscious experience that gives rise to psychopharmacology, both recreational and therapeutic.

The human brain

The human brain is by far the most complex structure that we know of. It contains 100 billion neurones, each of which makes up to 10,000 synaptic connections, giving a total of more than 100 trillion synapses. It could almost be said that neurones must be produced at a mean rate of 4000 per second, and synapses formed at a rate of 40 million per second, during the nine months of human gestation. It has evolved over hundreds of millions of years but the dramatic forebrain and cortical development that makes us human has occurred relatively recently. Indeed the human brain has almost tripled in weight and volume to its present 1400 g and 1400 ml during the last 100,000 years. Almost all of this extra weight and volume is accounted for by cortex and almost all of this extra cortex is prefrontal cortex. In fact the prefrontal cortex represents 20% of total brain weight.

The blood–brain barrier

Our survival depends upon the brain's absolute needs for oxygen, glucose and homeostasis being met through the capillary network that supplies its blood.

The endothelial cells of this capillary network form the blood–brain barrier (BBB) (Fig. 3.1). These have tight junctions that bind adjacent endothelial cells together in a narrow band just below their apical surfaces. The endothelial cells of the capillary network therefore act like a membrane or sheath that is closely applied to the brain, both around it and within it. This sheath is itself sheathed by the foot

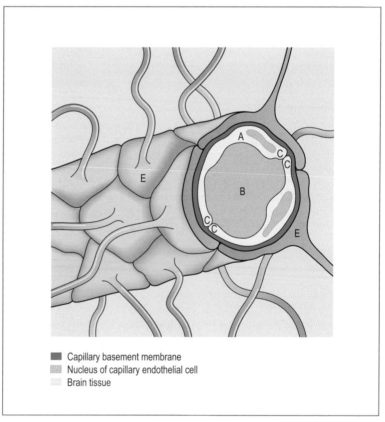

◼ Capillary basement membrane
▨ Nucleus of capillary endothelial cell
░ Brain tissue

Fig. 3.1 The blood–brain barrier. The blood–brain barrier consists of the endothelial cells (A) of the brain's capillaries (B) that are bound to each other at tight junctions (C), the capillary basement membrane and the foot processes of astrocytes (D) that are applied closely to the capillary basement membrane and to each other.

processes of astrocytes which thus essentially separate the capillaries of the brain from its neurones.

The BBB is both:

- a physical barrier that restricts the entrance of potentially harmful substances such as pathogens including bacteria and viruses, drugs including most antibiotics, immunoglobulins and even monoamine neurotransmitters and
- a system of cellular transport mechanisms that controls the entrance of essential nutrients such as sodium (Na^+) and potassium (K^+) ions, phenylalanine, methionine and glucose from the blood to the brain. The BBB maintains cerebral glucose levels at the expense of general blood glucose via a Na^+ linked active transport system.

Lipid-soluble substances such as ethanol and caffeine are able to diffuse across the BBB with relative ease. Lipid-soluble drugs also cross the BBB with ease but lipid-insoluble drugs pass into the brain very slowly. The BBB is therefore a significant consideration in the development of psychotropic drugs which of necessity must enter the brain. Various techniques are employed to circumvent it. Dopamine, for example, is an effective treatment for Parkinson's disease but it does not cross the BBB. However, L-dopa crosses it readily and is easily converted to dopamine (DA) in the brain.

Various factors increase the permeability of the BBB. These include ageing, hyperthermia, hypoxia, hypercapnia and head injury. Electro-convulsive therapy also increases the permeability of the BBB. The BBB is absent at the pituitary gland so that pituitary hormones may pass directly into the blood. It is also absent at the subfornical organ, a chemoreceptive area that controls water balance and has other homeostatic functions.

Neurones

The structural unit of the brain is the neurone (Fig. 3.2). A typical neurone consists of a cell body from which a single axon and many dendrites project. The axon divides into many terminal axon fibres. Neurones function by sending information to, and receiving information from, other neurones. This flow of information between neurones is made possible by chemical neurotransmission, the flow of neurotransmitters across the synapses between neurones. Information flow within neurones occurs by electrical neurotransmission.

Chemical neurotransmission is possible because the terminal axon fibres of one neurone, the presynaptic neurone, pass information to other neurones, the postsynaptic neurones, via synaptic connections at:

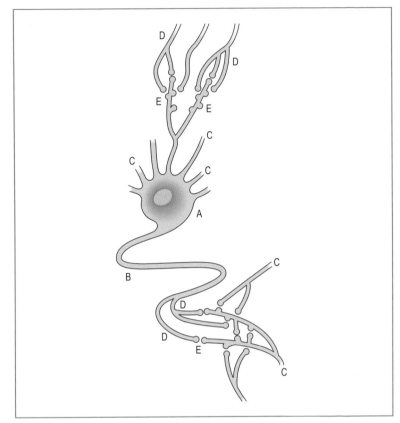

Fig. 3.2 A typical neurone. A neurone consists of a cell body (A) from which a single axon (B) and many dendrites (C) project. Presynaptic neurones pass information to postsynaptic neurones via synapses between their terminal axon fibres (D) and dendritic spines (E) on the dendrites of the postsynaptic neurone.

- their dendrites, usually at projections from them called dendritic spines
- their cell bodies and
- their terminal axon fibres.

In turn, postsynaptic neurones receive information from other neurones via synaptic connections at their dendrites/dendritic spines, cell bodies and terminal axon fibres. Given that almost all neurones both send and receive information it will be apparent that almost all are simultaneously both presynaptic and postsynaptic neurones.

The synapse

The functional unit of the brain is the synapse. Synapses are specialised junctions between neurones or between neurones and muscles or glands. A synapse consists of the presynaptic membrane of a terminal axon fibre from the presynaptic neurone, the postsynaptic membrane of the dendritic spine of the postsynaptic neurone and the narrow (10–50 nm) synaptic cleft between them (Fig. 3.3).

The brain and glucose

The brain accounts for only 2% of our bodyweight but it receives 15% of our cardiac output and utilises 20% of the oxygen and 10% of the energy that we consume. It has stores of glucose and glycogen sufficient for only a few minutes of normal metabolism and it is therefore completely dependent upon glucose supplied by the blood.

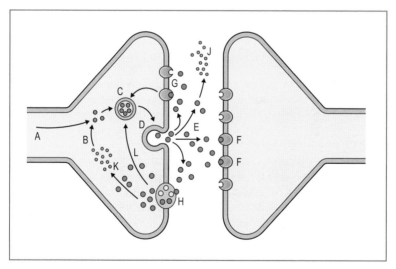

Fig. 3.3 A synapse. Neurotransmitter is synthesised in either the cell body of the neurone from where it is transported down the axon (A) or the terminal axon fibres (B). It is stored in synaptic vesicles (C). When the terminal axon fibre depolarises, synaptic vesicles fuse with the presynaptic membrane (D) and release neurotransmitter into the synapse (E). Once in the synapse, neurotransmitter either binds to receptors on the postsynaptic membrane (F), binds to autoreceptors on the presynaptic membrane (G) or on the cell body of the presynaptic neurone, binds to reuptake transporter proteins on the presynaptic membrane (H) or is inactivated by catabolic enzymes in the synapse (J). Neurotransmitter that re-enters the presynaptic neurone via reuptake transporter proteins is either inactivated by catabolic enzymes (K) or stored again in synaptic vesicles (L).

Adenosine triphosphate (ATP) is produced in the brain as in all other tissues by oxidative phosphorylation of glucose. In addition however, and in contrast to almost all other tissues, approximately 10% of the brain's glucose is converted to glutamate, gamma-amino butyric acid (GABA) and aspartate – the so-called glutamate group of amino acids – via the glutamate–GABA shunt. This utilises the enzyme glutamate decarboxylase to catalyse the conversion of glutamate, produced by the Krebs cycle, to GABA. Glutamate, GABA and aspartate are neurotransmitters that together account for 75% of the free amino acids in the brain.

Neurotransmission

Neurotransmission may be defined as the conversion of an action potential in the presynaptic neurone into a chemical messenger, the neurotransmitter (see Box 3.1), that is capable of crossing the synapse and eliciting a change at the postsynaptic neurone. Neurotransmission may be considered under the headings of presynaptic, synaptic and postsynaptic events.

Presynaptic events

The key presynaptic events are the synthesis and storage of neurotransmitter and its release into the synapse. Some psychotropic drugs exert their effect by modifying neurotransmitter synthesis, storage or release.

Neurotransmitter synthesis

The enzymes necessary for neurotransmitter synthesis are proteins which are produced in the cell body of the presynaptic neurone because they are coded for by genes in its nucleus. These enzymes synthesise neurotransmitter both in the cell body, from where it is transported to

---

Box 3.1: Definition of a neurotransmitter

A neurotransmitter may be defined as a substance that:

- is synthesised in the presynaptic neurone
- is stored inactively in synaptic vesicles in the terminal axon fibres
- is released from the synaptic vesicles into the synapse
- binds to receptors on the dendritic spines of the postsynaptic neurone
- binds to receptors on the presynaptic neurone
- binds to reuptake transporter proteins on the presynaptic membrane and
- is degraded and rendered inactive by specific enzyme systems in the synapse and terminal axon fibres

the terminal axon fibres, and in the terminal axon fibres themselves. Neuropeptides (see below) are an exception to this general principle in that they are only produced in the cell body because they are coded for by genes in its nucleus. Once synthesised, neuropeptides are transported to the terminal axon fibres.

Neurotransmitter storage

Neurotransmitter is stored in synaptic vesicles in the terminal axon fibres (Fig. 3.3). It is actively pumped into these vesicles by a transporter protein. Small molecule neurotransmitters such as monoamines (see below) are stored in vesicles that are <100 nm in diameter. Large molecule neurotransmitters such as neuropeptides (see below) are stored in vesicles that are 100–250 nm in diameter. Synaptic vesicles themselves are stored close to the presynaptic membrane, either anchored to the neuronal cytoskeleton or to the presynaptic membrane itself.

Neurotransmitter release

The release of neurotransmitter into the synapse depends on the influx of calcium ions (Ca^{2+}) into the presynaptic neurone. The evidence to support this view is that:

- low- or high-voltage Ca^{2+} ion channels that are embedded in the presynaptic membrane open when the presynaptic neurone depolarises
- Ca^{2+} concentration increases in the presynaptic neurone when it depolarises because Ca^{2+} influx from the synapse occurs
- Ca^{2+} promotes neurotransmitter synthesis (see above) by enzyme activation and
- Ca^{2+} facilitates the fusion of synaptic vesicles with the presynaptic membrane.

Neurotransmitter is released into the synapse by exocytosis following fusion of synaptic vesicles with the presynaptic membrane. The empty synaptic vesicle is recycled following exocytosis.

Synaptic events

Once released into the synapse neurotransmitters may:

- bind to receptors on the postsynaptic membrane (see below)
- bind to autoreceptors on the presynaptic membrane or on the cell body of the presynaptic neurone
- bind to reuptake transporter proteins on the presynaptic membrane or
- be inactivated by catabolic enzymes.

Some psychotropic drugs exert their effect by activation or inhibition of presynaptic autoreceptors, by inhibition of reuptake transporter proteins or by inhibition of catabolic enzymes.

Autoreceptors

Neurotransmitters generally exert an inhibitory effect on further neurotransmitter release when they bind to receptors referred to as autoreceptors on the presynaptic membrane. For example, noradrenaline (NA; norepinephrine) released into the synapse binds not only to postsynaptic $\alpha1$ and $\beta1$ noradrenergic receptors but also to $\alpha2$ autoreceptors on the presynaptic membrane. This $\alpha2$ binding inhibits presynaptic depolarisation and brings neurotransmitter release to an end. Neurotransmitters also bind to receptors referred to as somatodendritic autoreceptors on the cell body of the presynaptic neurone. For example, NA binds to somatodendritic $\alpha2$ autoreceptors. Such binding also inhibits presynaptic depolarisation and brings neurotransmitter release to an end.

Reuptake transporter proteins

Neurotransmitter in the synapse binds to specific reuptake transporter proteins on the presynaptic membrane. These return the neurotransmitter to the terminal axon fibres where it is either stored in a synaptic vesicle for subsequent re-release or degraded by catabolic enzymes and recycled.

The most important reuptake transporter proteins from a psychopharmacological perspective are those for DA, NA and serotonin (5HT) and many AD drugs act by inhibiting these, thus increasing synaptic neurotransmitter concentrations and neurotransmitter binding to the postsynaptic membrane.

Catabolic enzymes

Neurotransmitter is degraded and rendered inactive by specific enzyme systems located in the synapse and in the terminal axon fibres. Acetylcholine (Ach), for example, is inactivated by acetylcholinesterase in the synapse which mediates its hydrolysis to acetate and choline. NA on the other hand is inactivated by catechol-O-methyl-transferase (COMT) in the synapse and, following reuptake via the reuptake transporter proteins, by monoamine oxidase (MAO) in the mitochondria of the terminal axon fibre. Neuropeptides are degraded by catabolic peptidases located in the synapse.

The most important catabolic enzymes from a psychopharmacological perspective are MAO and acetylcholinesterase. Some antidepressant (AD) drugs act by inhibiting the former while most drugs for the treatment of Alzheimer's disease act by inhibiting the latter.

Postsynaptic events

The primary function of neurotransmitters released into the synapse is to bind to receptors on the postsynaptic membrane. The effect of neurotransmitter/receptor binding, and the speed with which it occurs, depends on the type of receptor involved as follows:

- Ionotropic (or ligand gated) receptors are ion channels that open when their neurotransmitter binds to them. Such ion channel opening may
  - allow Na^+ ion influx in which case an immediate (within 1–2 milliseconds) excitatory postsynaptic potential (EPSP) or depolarisation occurs, for example when Ach binds to nicotinic receptors of the neuromuscular junction (see below), or
  - allow chloride (Cl^-) ion influx in which case an immediate (within 1–2 milliseconds) inhibitory postsynaptic potential (IPSP) or hyperpolarisation occurs, for example when GABA binds to the $GABA_A$ receptor (see below).
- Guanine triphosphate or G-protein coupled (or metabotropic) receptors. These do not function as ion channels and neurotransmitter/receptor binding instead causes activation of the G-protein which, either directly or indirectly, causes opening of separate ion channels in the postsynaptic neurone. Ion channels opened by G-protein coupled receptors may cause
  - an EPSP and depolarisation, for example when nicotine binds to the muscarinic cholinergic receptor, or
  - an IPSP and hyperpolarisation, for example when GABA binds to the $GABA_B$ receptor (see below).

The term nonsynaptic diffusion neurotransmission has been coined to describe neurotransmission that occurs between neurones because neurotransmitters diffuse from the synapse into which they are released to a more distant postsynaptic neurone where they exert an excitatory or inhibitory effect.

Neurotransmitters

A practical classification of the most important neurotransmitters is presented in Table 3.1. The most important neurotransmitters from a psychopharmacological perspective are the catecholamines DA and NA, the indolanine 5HT, Ach, the amino acids GABA and glutamate and the neuronally synthesised gas, nitric oxide (NO). These will be discussed in some detail below. Some other neurotransmitters will be commented upon briefly.

Neurotransmitters may also be classified by their size. Thus small molecule (or simple or classical) neurotransmitters include dopamine, noradrenaline (norepinephrine), serotonin, acetylcholine, GABA and glutamate while large (or complex) molecule neurotransmitters include the neuropeptides such as β-endorphin. Cotransmission or colocalisation refers to the observation that small and large molecule neurotransmitters may be released from the same neurone, for example DA with cholecystokinin (CCK) (see Box 3.2). The mechanisms by which cotransmitters interact and the purpose of cotransmission are not yet fully understood.

Box 3.2: Dale's principle

The British physiologist Sir Henry Hallet Dale (1875–1968) shared the Nobel Prize in Physiology or Medicine in 1936 with the Austrian Otto Loewi (1873–1961) for their discoveries about the chemical nature of neurotransmission. Dale also developed the system of naming neurones by the neurotransmitter they release. Thus, neurones releasing noradrenaline (NA) are noradrenergic neurones while those releasing serotonin (5HT) are serotonergic neurones.

Dale's principle states that every neurone releases only one type of neurotransmitter. This principle is now known to be incorrect and it has been demonstrated that many neurones release more than one neurotransmitter, usually a small molecule such as a monoamine or an amino acid along with a large molecule such as a neuropeptide (Bear et al, 2001). This phenomenon is referred to as cotransmission or colocalisation.

Dopamine

Dopaminergic systems

The three dopaminergic systems of most importance to psychopharmacology originate in the midbrain and diencephalon and are depicted in Figure 3.4.

The mesocorticolimbic system

Dopaminergic neurones project from the ventral tegmental area to the limbic (amygdala and nucleus accumbens/ventral striatum), septal and frontocortical (prefrontal and anterior cingulate) areas. The principal functions of DA in health and disease are as follows:

- frontal DA D_1 receptors appear to play an important role in normal cognitive function

Table 3.1: A practical classification of the most important neurotransmitters

Neurotransmitter class	Neurotransmitter
Amines	Dopamine (DA), a catecholamine Noradrenaline (NA), a catecholamine Serotonin (5HT), an indolamine Acetylcholine (Ach)
Amino acids	Gamma aminobutyric acid (GABA) Glutamate Aspartate Glycine
Neuronally synthesised gases	Nitric oxide (NO) Carbon monoxide (CO)
Opioid peptides	β Endorphin Methionine-encephalin Leucine-encephalin
Hormones	Hypothalamic hormones • corticotrophin release hormone (CRH) • tyrotrophin release hormone (TRH) • somatostatin Pituitary hormones • growth hormone (GH) • thyroid stimulating hormone (TSH) • corticotrophin (ACTH) • vasopressin Gastrointestinal hormones • cholecystokinin (CCK) • vasoactive intestinal peptide (VIP) Circulating hormones • angiotensin • insulin • leptin

- the mesocorticolimbic system is involved in reward and pleasure, drugs of abuse such as nicotine, alcohol, opiates, cocaine and amfetamine causing release of DA at the nucleus accumbens
- excess mesocorticolimbic dopaminergic function may underpin schizophrenia, especially its positive symptoms, because all antipsychotic (AP) drugs are mesolimbic DA D_2 receptor antagonists
- deficient mesocorticolimbic dopaminergic function in the prefrontal and cingulate cortex has been implicated in the negative symptoms of schizophrenia while

- mesocorticolimbic dopaminergic dysfunction has been implicated in mood disorders, particularly depression (prefrontal cortex/cingulate gyrus, nucleus accumbens), and in psychomotor retardation (dorsolateral prefrontal cortex, caudate nucleus).

The nigrostriatal system

Dopaminergic neurones project from the zona compacta of the substantia nigra to the striatum. Degeneration of this system causes Parkinson's disease while blockade of DA D_2 receptors here by AP drugs causes extrapyramidal syndromes such as dystonia, akathisia and Parkinsonism. Supersensitivity of nigrostriatal DA D_2 receptors caused by AP drugs may be implicated in tardive dyskinesia.

The tuberoinfundibular system

Dopaminergic neurones project from the arcuate nucleus of the hypothalamus to the pituitary gland. DA inhibits the release of prolactin and blockade of DA D_2 receptors here by AP drugs causes hyperprolactinaemia.

Biochemistry and receptors

DA is synthesised from phenylalanine via L-tyrosine and degraded by MAO and COMT to homovanillic acid (HVA).

DA receptors are subdivided into the D_1 like G_S coupled ($D_{1 \& 5}$) and the D_2 like G_1 coupled ($D_{2, 3 \& 4}$) classes (see below).

Clinical psychopharmacology

All AP drugs are potent D_2 receptor antagonists (and many are also potent $5HT_{2A}$ receptor antagonists). The exact anatomical location of the therapeutic effect of AP drugs is as yet unclear, but improvements in positive and negative symptoms are thought to result from altered dopaminergic function in the limbic and prefrontal cortex respectively.

Tricyclic (TCA) AD drugs inhibit the reuptake of DA to the presynaptic neurone by the DA transporter protein while monoamine Type A oxidase inhibitor (MAOI) AD drugs increase synaptic DA by inhibiting MAO, its catabolic enzyme.

Amfetamines increase synaptic DA by causing its release into the synapse and both amfetamines and cocaine potently inhibit the DA reuptake transporter protein.

Noradrenaline (norepinephrine)

Noradrenergic systems

Noradrenergic neurones originate in the locus coeruleus in the floor of the 4th ventricle in the brainstem (Fig. 3.4). They project throughout the brain but especially to the medulla and spinal cord, the cerebellum,

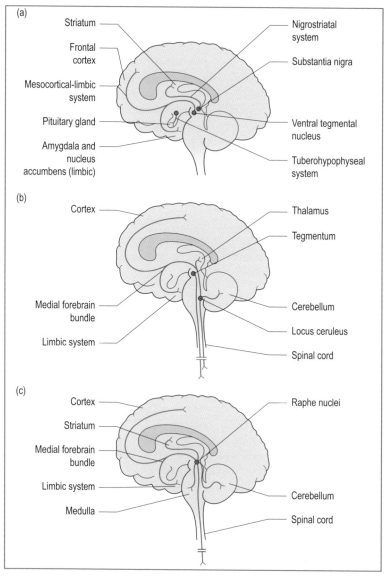

Fig. 3.4 Schematic representation. (**a**) The mesocorticolimbic and nigrostriatal dopaminergic systems originate in the midbrain and project to the frontal cortex and limbic system, and to the striatum, respectively. The tuberohypophyseal dopaminergic system originates in the diencephalon and projects to the pituitary gland. (**b**) Noradrenergic neurones originating in the locus ceruleus project to the cortex, limbic system, thalamus, cerebellum and spinal cord. Tegmental noradrenergic neurones project to the brainstem and spinal cord. (**c**) Serotonergic neurones arise in the raphe nuclei and project to the cortex, limbic system, striatum, cerebellum, medulla and spinal cord.

the limbic system and thalamus, and the cortex. Noradrenergic systems are believed to be critical to arousal, attention, mood and pain because:

- activity in noradrenergic neurones in the locus coeruleus increases in response to novel or aversive stimuli
- α_1 and α_2 receptor antagonists cause sedation
- many antidepressant drugs increase noradrenergic neurotransmission and
- AD drugs that increase synaptic NA concentrations are effective treatments for some pain syndromes.

Biochemistry and receptors

NA is synthesised from phenylalanine (via dopamine) and degraded by MAO and COMT to 3-methoxy-4-hydroxy phenylglycol and 3-methoxy-4-hydroxy mandelic acid respectively.

Noradrenergic receptor subtypes include $\alpha_{1\ \&\ 2}$ and β_{1-3} (see below).

Clinical psychopharmacology

Abnormalities of noradrenergic function are believed to play a role in depression and bipolar disorder. TCA AD drugs such as desipramine and nortriptyline (secondary amines) increase synaptic NA by inhibiting its reuptake to the presynaptic neurone by the NA transporter protein. The TCA AD drugs amitriptyline and impiramine (tertiary amines) behave similarly but less potently than secondary amines and they also inhibit the 5HT reuptake transporter (see below).

MAOI AD drugs increase synaptic NA by inhibiting MAO, its catabolic enzyme. There are two types of MAO, MAO-A and MAO-B. MAO-A is the most efficient in degrading NA (and 5HT) and its irreversible inhibition by MAOIs (especially phenelzine) may impair the metabolism of both dietary tyramine and sympathomimetic drugs such as phenylpropanolamine, leading to severe hypertension. Moclobemide is a reversible inhibitor of MAO-A and it poses much less of a risk in this regard.

Amfetamines increase synaptic NA by promoting its rapid release into the synapse and both amfetamines and cocaine potently inhibit the NA reuptake transporter.

Serotonin

Serotonergic systems

Serotonergic neurones originate in the dorsal and median raphe nucleii in the brainstem (Fig. 3.4). They project throughout the brain but especially to the medulla and spinal cord, the cerebellum, the limbic system and striatum, and the cortex. Serotonergic systems are believed to be critical to sleep, appetite and mood because:

* reduced serotonergic function may cause insomnia and depression
* enhanced serotonergic function may cause appetite reduction and weight loss and
* most AD drugs increase serotonergic neurotransmission.

Biochemistry and receptors

5HT is synthesised from tryptophan and degraded by MAO to 5-hydroxyindolacetic acid.

Serotonergic receptor subtypes include $5HT_{1A-1F}$, $5HT_{2A-2C}$, $5HT_3$, $5HT_4$, $5HT_{5A-5C}$, $5HT_6$ and $5HT_7$.

Clinical psychopharmacology

Abnormalities of serotonergic function are believed to be important in depression, anxiety, psychosis (many AP drugs are potent $5HT_{2A}$ receptor antagonists) and nausea (5HT reuptake inhibitor AD drugs cause nausea while ondansetron, a potent $5HT_3$ receptor antagonist, is an effective antiemetic). Selective 5HT reuptake inhibitor (SSRI) AD drugs such as fluoxetine and paroxetine increase synaptic 5HT by inhibiting its reuptake to the presynaptic neurone by the 5HT transporter protein. TCA AD drugs such as amitriptyline and impiramine (tertiary amines) have a similar effect and most TCA AD drugs also cause release of 5HT into the synapse. MAOI AD drugs increase synaptic 5HT by inhibiting MAO, its catabolic enzyme.

Amfetamines increase synaptic 5HT by causing its release into the synapse while lysergic acid diethylamine (LSD) and psilocybin are $5HT_{1A}$ and $5HT_{2A \ \& \ 2C}$ partial agonists.

Acetylcholine

Cholinergic systems

Ach is best known as the primary neurotransmitter in the peripheral nervous system but it also plays a critical role in the central nervous system where cholinergic neurones project from the septal nucleii and nucleus basalis of Meynert in the ventromedial globus pallidus, to the hippocampus, amygdala and thalamus, and throughout the cortex. Cholinergic neurones appear to be critical to memory because they degenerate in dementia. Cholinergic neurones also project from the brainstem to the basal ganglia, where many cholinergic interneurones occur. These play a role in the modulation of movement.

Biochemistry and receptors

Ach is synthesised from acetyl-CoA and choline by the enzyme choline acetyl transferase and degraded by acetylcholinesterase to acetic acid and choline.

Cholinergic receptors may be nicotinic (rapidly acting, excitatory, ion channel receptors – see below) or muscarinic (slowly acting, excitatory or inhibitory, G-protein coupled receptors – see below). Nicotinic receptors occur at the neuromuscular junction and at other sites including the brain while muscarinic receptors, of which there are five subtypes, M_{1-5}, occur in the brain and in cardiac and smooth muscle.

Clinical psychopharmacology

Many drugs used in psychiatry have potent anticholinergic or atropine-like effects and may cause dry mouth, increased sweating, blurred vision, constipation and urinary retention. Cholinergic agonists tend to cause tremor and anticholinergic/antimuscarinic drugs are given to overcome the rigidity and bradykinesia of both idiopathic and iatrogenic Parkinsonism. Dysfunction of M_1 receptors, which are always excitatory, has been implicated in dementia while dysfunction of M_2 receptors, which are always inhibitory, has been implicated in mania. Acetylcholinesterase inhibitors such as donepezil may slow cognitive decline in dementia.

Nicotine, acting on cortical nicotinic receptors, increases cortical Ach. Anticholinergic/antimuscarinic drugs induce a sense of euphoria and are frequently misused. It has also been reported that they are administered to terrorists by their leaders because they facilitate brainwashing and induce a sense of invulnerability in suicide bombers (Radio Free Europe, 2004).

Gamma-amino butyric acid

GABA-ergic systems

GABA, the main inhibitory neurotransmitter in the brain, is found in the substantia nigra, striatum (caudate, putamen and globus pallidus) and hypothalamus as well as in the cerebellum (Purkinje cells) and spinal cord.

Biochemistry and receptors

GABA is synthesised from glutamate via the GABA shunt and degraded to succinic acid.

GABA receptors are subdivided into $GABA_A$ (ion channel receptors that are widely distributed in the brain) and $GABA_B$ (G-protein coupled receptors that are less widely distributed in the brain) classes.

Clinical psychopharmacology

Loss of GABA neurones in the striatum occurs in Huntington's chorea. GABA dysfunction has been implicated in both anxiety and epilepsy because benzodiazepine (BZD) drugs, potent $GABA_A$ receptor agonists, are very effective anxiolytic and antiepileptic drugs. Baclofen, used to reduce severe spasticity of voluntary muscles, is a potent presynaptic $GABA_B$ receptor agonist.

Alcohol enhances GABA-ergic function and changes at the $GABA_A$ receptor are thought to be involved in alcohol tolerance and dependence.

Glutamate

Glutamate and aspartate are the major excitatory neurotransmitters throughout the brain. Glutamate binds to either:

- ion channel or ionotropic (N-methyl, D-aspartate or NMDA, alpha-amino-3-hydroxy-5-methyl-4-isoxazole propionic acid or AMPA, kainate or K and quisqualate or Q) receptors or to
- metabotropic (G-protein coupled or mGluR) receptors.

There are six subtypes of metabotropic glutamate receptors. These are necessary for long-term potentiation (or prolonged efficacy of a network of synapses, a process that may be involved in learning because blockade of NMDA receptors inhibits learning) in the hippocampus and may be involved in memory. Glutamate biding at the NMDA receptor permits Ca^{2+} influx which causes long-term potentiation via a cascade of biochemical steps.

Clinical psychopharmacology

Despite its critical physiological role, glutamate is a potent neurotoxin that causes neuronal death via excessive stimulation and excessive Ca^{2+} influx. Excessive NMDA receptor stimulation is thought to underlie the pathophysiology of stroke, head injury and epilepsy. This has led to efforts to develop NMDA antagonists such as lamotrigine (which inhibits glutamate release and is an effective antiepileptic drug) and memantine (an NMDA receptor antagonist that is licensed for the treatment of dementia). Phencyclidine and ketamine are both antagonists of the NMDA receptor. These drugs are psychotomimetic and there is increasing evidence for glutaminergic dysfunction in schizophrenia.

Nitric oxide

The Americans Robert Furchgott (1916 to present), Louis Ignarro (1941 to present) and Ferid Murad (1936 to present) shared the Nobel Prize in Physiology or Medicine in 1998 for discovering that NO is a signalling molecule in the cardiovascular system. Signal transmission by a gas produced by one cell and that then diffuses to other cells and regulates their function is an entirely new biological paradigm.

Biochemistry and receptors

The enzyme NO synthetase is present in endothelial cells and some neurones where it converts L-arginine to NO and L-citrulline. NO is not stored or released and does not bind to postsynaptic receptors. Rather it diffuses to other cells where it binds to guanylyl (or guanylate) cyclase and activates it. Guanylyl cyclase then catalyses the conversion of guanosine triphosphate (GTP) to 3,5-cyclic guanosine monophosphate (cGMP). Cyclic GMP is ultimately degraded to 5-guanosine monophosphate (5GMP) by phosphodiesterase enzymes, for example cGMP specific phosphodiesterase Type 5 (PDE-5) in the penis (see Fig. 13.1).

Clinical psychopharmacology

Endothelial NO diffuses to vascular smooth muscle causing relaxation and vasodilation. This is important to blood pressure regulation, gastrointestinal peristalsis and penile erection. Phosphodiesterase Type 5 inhibitors such as sildenafil promote the action of NO in the penis and are effective treatments for erectile impotence.

Opioid peptides

Opioid peptides include the endorphins and enkephalins and their β-endorphin, corticotrophin (ACTH), dynorphin/neo-endorphin and enkephalin precursors. Generally, opioid peptides are involved in mediating stress reactions, particularly pain, through their μ, δ and κ neuroreceptors. The β-endorphins are found almost exclusively within the hypothalamus. Enkephalins are more widely distributed in the brain and have been found in the striatum, limbic system including the amygdala, and in the periaqueductal grey matter.

Glycine

Glycine is second only to GABA as the most important inhibitory neurotransmitter in the brain. It is synthesised from serine and appears to modify the effects of glutamate and other excitatory amino acids by binding to NMDA receptors on neurones.

Substance P

A small family of three peptide neurotransmitters called neurokinins (NK) has recently been identified. The members of this family currently include Substance P, NK-A and NK-B. These are agonists at NK_1, NK_2 and NK_3 receptors respectively. Substance P is the main neurotransmitter within the substantia gelatinosa of the spinal cord where the dorsal root ganglion cells terminate and where it plays a role in the transmission of pain. It also appears to play a role in depression and NK_1 receptor antagonists are being investigated as potential antidepressant drugs. Curiously, the NK_1 receptor antagonists developed to date do not alleviate pain.

Neuroreceptors

Neurotransmitters cross the synapse and bind to neuroreceptors on the postsynaptic membrane. They are classified into 'superfamilies' of which the two most important are the ligand gated ion channel (ionotropic) receptors and the G-protein (metabotropic) coupled receptors. The principal neuroreceptors with their neurotransmitters and their effects are presented in Table 3.2. Tyrosine kinase-linked receptors are not yet of major importance to psychopharmacology.

Ligand gated ion channel (ionotropic) receptors

EPSP and depolarisation of the postsynaptic neurone depends on the opening of ion channels in the postsynaptic membrane and the subsequent influx of Na^+ ions and efflux of potassium (K^+) ions. IPSP and hyperpolarisation of the postsynaptic neurone on the other hand depend on the opening of ion channels in the postsynaptic membrane and the subsequent influx of both Cl^- and K^+ ions.

The ion channels responsible for ionic influx and efflux are the neuroreceptors for neurotransmitters such as Ach, GABA and glutamate. The response of a neurone to ion channel receptor activation by either the neurotransmitter (natural ligand) or a drug is rapid and brief. Two examples of ligand gated ion channel receptors are the $GABA_A$ receptor in the brain and the nicotinic receptor at the neuromuscular junction.

$GABA_A$ receptors

GABA is the main inhibitory neurotransmitter in the brain and is present at 40% of synapses. The $GABA_A$ receptor is composed of five cylinder-shaped protein subunits that are embedded parallel to each other across the cell membrane and that form a central channel that spans this membrane (see Fig. 11.1). This channel is approximately 0.5 nm in diameter in the absence of GABA and Cl^- ions are unable to pass through it. GABA induces conformational changes in the protein subunits when it binds to the $GABA_A$ receptor and the diameter of the

Table 3.2: Neuroreceptors with their neurotransmitters and their effects

Receptor superfamily	Receptor	Neurotransmitter	Effect
Ligand gated ion-channel (ionotropic)	$GABA_A$	GABA	Cl^- influx, IPSP
	Nicotinic	Acetylcholine	Na^+ influx, EPSP
	Glutamate NMDA, AMPA, K, Q	Glutamate	Ca^{2+} influx, EPSP
	Glycine	Glycine	Cl^- influx, IPSP
G-protein coupled (metabotropic)	Dopamine • $D_{1\,\&\,5}$ (G_S coupled) • $D_{2,\,3\,\&\,4}$ (G_i coupled)	Dopamine	• $D_{1\,\&\,5}$, adenylate cyclase activated • $D_{2,\,3\,\&\,4}$, adenylate cyclase inactivated
	Noradrenaline • $\alpha_{1\,\&\,2}$ • β_{1-3}	Noradrenaline	• α_1, K^+ influx, IPSP • α_2, K^+ influx, IPSP • β_{1-3}, adenylate cyclase activated
	Serotonin • $5HT_{1A-1F}$ • $5HT_{2A-2C}$ • $5HT_3$ • $5HT_4$ • $5HT_{5A-5C}$ • $5HT_6$ • $5HT_7$	Serotonin	• $5HT_{1A}$, adenylate cyclase activated • $5HT_{1B}$, adenylate cyclase inactivated • $5HT_{1C\,\&\,2}$ phosphatidylinosital activated

Table 3.2: Neuroreceptors with their neurotransmitters and their effects—*cont'd*

Receptor superfamily	Receptor	Neurotransmitter	Effect
G-protein coupled (metabotropic)	$GABA_B$	GABA	IPSP
	Muscarinic • $M_{1\&3}$ (G_S coupled) • M_2 (G_i coupled)	Acetylcholine	• $M_{1\&3}$, Ca^{2+} influx, EPSP • M_2, K^+ influx, IPSP
	Glutamate • $mGluR_{1-5}$	Glutamate	EPSP
	Cannabinoid • CB_1 • CB_2	Endocannabinoid	See text
Tyrosine kinase linked	Nerve growth factor (NGF)	–	–
	Neurotrophins	–	–

channel increases to 3 nm. Cl^- ions now readily pass through it into the postsynaptic neurone where they induce an IPSP and hyperpolarisation.

BZD drugs such as diazepam have high affinity for, and are agonists at, the $GABA_A$ receptor. $GABA_A$ receptors possess two binding sites, one for GABA, the natural ligand, on the α protein subunit and the other for BZD drugs on the β protein subunit. Binding of a BZD drug such as diazepam to the $GABA_A$ receptor enhances the effect of GABA and causes a greater influx of Cl^- than is possible through binding of GABA alone. This is an example of allosteric modulation.

Nicotinic receptors

Like the $GABA_A$ receptor, the cholinergic nicotinic receptor of the neuromuscular junction consists of five protein subunits that form a channel across the cell membrane. This channel opens when Ach binds to the α subunit and the subsequent influx of Na^+ ions causes an EPSP and depolarisation.

Glutamate receptors behave similarly to nicotinic receptors in that they elicit an EPSP at NMDA, AMPA, K and Q receptors.

G-protein coupled (metabotropic) receptors

Many receptors are not ion channels themselves but are linked to ion channels and to enzyme systems by guanine triphosphate binding, or G, proteins (Fig. 3.5). Such G-protein coupled or metabotropic receptors have seven protein subunits that span the cell membrane. The amino acid sequence joining, for example, the 5th and the 6th subunits of the G-protein, and that extending from the 7th subunit into the cytoplasm, are highly variable and form the site at which the receptor is coupled with the G-protein. The G-protein itself is embedded in the intracellular or cytoplasmic surface of the cell membrane. The shape of these amino acid sequences is distorted when the ligand binds to the receptor and this distortion activates the G-protein. Activated G-protein in turn either stimulates (G_S at the β_2 adrenergic receptor for example) or inhibits (G_I at the α_1 adrenergic receptor for example) adenylate cyclase or other 'second messengers'. G-protein modulation of adenylate cyclase activity is slow and prolonged, a fact that may explain the delayed onset of action but prolonged effect of some psychotropic drugs.

Examples of G-protein coupled receptors include:

- dopaminergic receptors (D_1 like G_S coupled and D_2 like G_I coupled)
- adrenergic receptors that bind catecholamines ($\alpha_{1\ \&\ 2}$, β_{1-3})
- serotonergic receptors ($5HT_{1A-1F}$, $5HT_2$)
- GABA receptors ($GABA_B$)

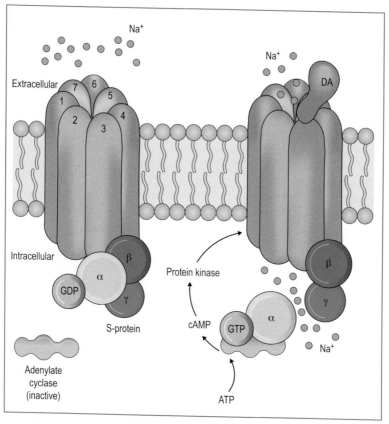

Fig. 3.5 Schematic of the dopamine D_1 receptor, a G-protein coupled receptor. The dopamine D_1 receptor has 7 protein subunits that form an ion channel. The extracellular sections of the 3rd and 5th protein subunits form the dopamine binding site while the intracellular section of the 3rd forms the G-protein binding site. The G-protein consists of α, β and γ subunits of which the α subunit normally binds guanine diphosphate (GDP). When dopamine binds to the 3rd and 5th protein subunits of the receptor, the α subunit loses GDP and binds guanine triphosphate (GTP). The α subunit/GTP complex then dissociates from the β and γ subunits and binds with adenylate cyclase, activating it. Activated adenylate cyclase converts adenosine triphosphate (ATP) to cyclic adenosine 3,5-monophosphate (cAMP) which then activates protein kinase. Protein kinase in turn phosphorylates the ion channel allowing influx of Na^+ ions which causes an excitatory postsynaptic potential.

- muscarinic cholinergic receptors (M_{1-3})
- glutamate receptors ($mGLUr_{1-5}$)
- cannabinoid receptors ($CB_{1\,\&\,2}$)
- melatonin receptors (MT_1 and MT_2).

It will be seen that all neuropeptides and many important small molecule neurotransmitters – DA, NA, 5HT and glutamate – bind to G-protein coupled receptors. Indeed all of the neuroreceptors that are currently important to psychopharmacology, with the exception of the ion channel $GABA_A$ and the glutamate receptors, are G-protein coupled. Two examples of G-protein coupled receptors are DA D_1 and the cannabinoid $CB_{1 \& 2}$ neuroreceptors.

Dopamine D_1 receptors

The DA D_1 receptor is a good example of a G-protein coupled or metabotropic receptor (see Fig. 3.5). It consists of 446 amino acids that form seven cylinder-shaped protein subunits that are embedded parallel to each other across the cell membrane. The extracellular ends of these subunits, particularly the 3rd and 5th, form the binding site for DA while the intracellular end of the 3rd subunit forms the binding site for the G-protein.

G-proteins are made up of α, β and γ subunits of which the α subunit can bind either guanine diphosphate (GDP) or guanine triphosphate (GTP). The G-protein is inactive when GDP is bound to the α subunit. However, when GTP binds to it, the α subunit/GTP complex dissociates from the β and γ subunits and binds with adenylate cyclase, activating it. The α subunit/GTP complex dissociates during this process, the α subunit subsequently reuniting with the β and γ subunits of the G-protein.

Activated adenylate cyclase converts ATP to cyclic adenosine 3,5 monophosphate (cyclic AMP or cAMP) which then activates protein kinase. Protein kinase in turn phosphorylates an ion channel allowing an influx of Na^+ ions which causes an EPSP and depolarisation.

The DA D_2 receptor functions in a manner that is similar to the DA D_1 receptor. However, activation of the G-protein in the case of the D_2 receptor inhibits adenylate cyclase (G_I at the α_1 adrenergic receptor for example).

Cannabinoid receptors

Investigation of the opiates, drugs that had been used for therapeutic and recreational purposes for millennia, led to the discovery of the opiate neuroreceptors (μ, σ and κ) and the endogenous opioid peptides such as β endorphin. More recently, investigation of cannabis, another drug that had been used for therapeutic and recreational purposes for millennia, led to the discovery of two cannabinoid neuroreceptors ($CB_{1 \& 2}$) and five endogenous cannabinoids or endocannabinoids, for example anandamide. The CB_1 receptor is present in the basal ganglia, cerebellum, hippocampus and cortex while the CB_2 receptor is present in peripheral nerve terminals and other peripheral tissues.

Rimonabant, a selective CB_1 receptor antagonist, has shown efficacy in the treatment of obesity and in smoking cessation. It has not shown efficacy in schizophrenia. Other potential uses of CB_1 receptor antagonists include opiate and alcohol dependency, depression (increased prefrontal CB_1 receptor density has been reported in depressed suicide victims) and cognitive impairment.

Melatonin receptors

G-protein coupled melatonin MT_1 and MT_2 receptors occur in the suprachiasmatic nucleus. The agonist action of melatonin at these receptors is thought to induce sleep. Ramelteon, an MT_1 and MT_2 receptor agonist, has recently been approved in the US for the treatment of insomnia (see Chapter 11).

References and further reading

Bear MF, Conners BW, Paradisa MA (2001) Neuroscience: Exploring the Brain. Baltimore, Lippincott, pp. 78–99.

Hungund BL, Vinod KY, Kassir SA et al (2004) Upregulation of CB1 receptors and agonist-stimulated [^{35}S]GTPgammaS binding in the prefrontal cortex of depressed suicide victims. Molecular Psychiatry 9(2):184–190.

Lingford-Hughes A (2004) Clinical neuroanatomy. In: Core Psychiatry (Eds Wright P, Phelan M and Stern J) (2nd Edition). London, Elsevier Saunders, pp. 13–34.

Radio Free Europe (2004) Inside Iraq available at http://www.rferl.org/reports/iraq-report/2004/03/11-260304.asp (accessed May 2005).

Stahl SM (2000) Principles of chemical neurotransmission. In: Essential Psychopharmacology – Neuroscientific Basis and Practical Applications (2nd Edition). Cambridge, Cambridge University Press, 33 pp.

Wright P (2004) Psychopharmacology. In: Core Psychiatry (Eds Wright P, Phelan M and Stern J) (2nd Edition). London, Elsevier Saunders, pp. 579–609.

4

Pharmacokinetics and pharmacodynamics of psychotropic drugs

Introduction

Pharmacokinetics may be succinctly described as the study of the effects of the body on a drug. Pharmacodynamics may be similarly described as the study of the effects of a drug on the body.

Pharmacokinetics

Pharmacokinetics is the study of what happens to a drug and its metabolites in the body following administration by any route, and of how long this takes to happen. The pharmacokinetics of any drug ingested by an individual may therefore be described by consideration of how it is absorbed and what its bioavailability is, of how it is distributed within the body and of how it is metabolised and eliminated. It is important to appreciate that drugs are absorbed, distributed, metabolised and eliminated simultaneously.

Absorption

Absorption refers to the movement of a drug from its site of administration to the systemic circulation. Unless administered intravenously (IV), a drug must traverse several lipid-rich biological membranes before it reaches the systemic circulation. This is only possible when the drug is in solution. Absorption is achieved by the following four mechanisms:

- Passive diffusion – this depends on a concentration gradient between the site of administration of the drug and the systemic circulation. This gradient is very high immediately following administration and is initially maintained at a high level because drug entering the blood is quickly distributed throughout the body. The rate of diffusion decreases as the concentration of drug at the site of administration decreases and as its concentration in blood rises. Drugs that are lipid soluble, unionised and of low molecular weight diffuse most readily across biological membranes.

- Facilitated passive diffusion – this is similar to passive diffusion in that it depends on a concentration gradient but differs in that diffusion is facilitated by carrier molecules. Carrier molecules only transport specific substrates and their supply is limited. Facilitated passive diffusion therefore exhibits both selectivity and saturability.

- Active transport – this depends on carrier molecules so it also exhibits selectivity and saturability. It differs from facilitated passive diffusion in that it utilises energy and can transport molecules against a concentration gradient.

- Pinocytosis – this energy-dependent process is the means by which protein drugs are absorbed.

Orally administered drugs

Psychotropic drugs are most often administered orally, less often intra-muscularly (IM) and only occasionally IV. Orally administered drugs are absorbed in the stomach and proximal small intestine. The rate of absorption depends on factors such as the disintegration of the tablet or capsule, the ease with which the drug enters solution, its physico-chemical properties in the presence of hydrochloric acid, its lipid solubility, whether the stomach is empty (this generally facilitates absorption) or full (this generally delays absorption) and concomitant treatment with other drugs that delay gastric emptying, for example tricyclic antidepressant (AD) drugs which have marked anticholinergic activity. The absorption of drugs that dissolve slowly and/or have poor lipophilicity is dependent on them spending sufficient time in the gastrointestinal tract. Rapid intestinal transit caused by diarrhoea or other drugs may therefore greatly impair absorption.

Orally administered drugs are initially absorbed more rapidly than they are eliminated with the result that the plasma level of the drug gradually increases. The peak plasma level or C_{MAX} is reached when the rates of absorption and elimination are equal, and the time taken to reach this point is referred to as T_{MAX}. The plasma level of the drug falls following C_{MAX} because the rate of elimination increasingly exceeds that of absorption.

The time taken for the plasma level of a drug to fall to half of any given value is referred to as its half-life or $T_{1/2}$ (Fig. 4.1). For almost all drugs, with the important exception of phenytoin, $T_{1/2}$ is constant. For example a plasma drug level of 100 ng/ml will drop to 50 ng/ml after one $T_{1/2}$, to 25 ng/ml after a further $T_{1/2}$, and to 12.5 ng/ml after a third $T_{1/2}$. It will be apparent that plasma drug level will effectively drop to zero and the drug will be eliminated from the body after 4 or 5 half-lives (4–$5 \times T_{1/2}$) have passed.

Parenterally administered drugs

Drugs administered by the IM route are rapidly absorbed and enter the systemic circulation quickly. They thus achieve higher peak plasma levels faster (higher C_{MAX} and shorter T_{MAX}) than the same dose of the same drug administered orally (Fig. 4.1).

Drugs administered by the IV route enter the systemic circulation immediately. This route also ensures 100% bioavailability (see below).

Steady state

It will be appreciated that second and subsequent doses of a drug increase the plasma level already achieved by a first dose. With continued dosing the rate at which drug enters the body eventually comes to equal the rate at which it is removed from the body and a relatively constant plasma level is achieved. This is referred to as

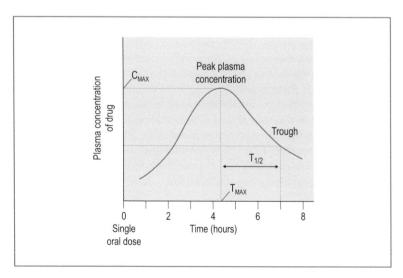

Fig. 4.1 A diagram of peak plasma concentration (C_{MAX}), the time taken to reach peak plasma concentration (T_{MAX}) and the half-life ($T_{1/2}$) of a drug (single oral dose of drug administered at time 0).

steady state. In the same way that it takes $4\text{--}5 \times T_{1/2}$ to eliminate a drug from the body it also takes $4\text{--}5 \times T_{1/2}$ to achieve steady state with continued dosing.

Bioavailability

It is important to differentiate between absorption of a drug from the gastrointestinal tract and the availability of that drug in the systemic circulation. Bioavailability refers to the proportion of a drug administered by any route that enters the systemic circulation. Bioavailability is 100% for IV administered drugs but for orally administered drugs it is always <100%. This is because:

- absorption from the gastrointestinal tract, even for the most lipid-soluble drug, is rarely 100% and/or because of
- first pass metabolism, the fact that a variable proportion of absorbed drug is metabolised in the gut lumen and wall and, much more significantly, while passing through the liver in the hepatic portal circulation.

The effect of incomplete absorption and/or first pass metabolism may range from insignificant to marked. It will be apparent that significant first pass metabolism will lead to the concentration of orally administered drug in the portal vein being significantly higher than that in the hepatic vein. This in turn explains why higher oral than IM doses of a drug may be required to achieve the same effect and why some drugs are ineffective if administered orally. For example oral administration of noradrenaline (NA; norepinephrine) is ineffective because first pass metabolism is virtually 100% and bioavailability is therefore 0%.

On the other hand bioavailability may be sufficient for therapeutic needs even when the rate of first pass metabolism of a drug is high if that metabolism produces an active metabolite. For example fluoxetine undergoes extensive first pass metabolism to norfluoxetine but norfluoxetine is as selective and as potent an inhibitor of the serotonin (5HT) reuptake transporter protein as fluoxetine.

Distribution

Once absorbed, a drug is distributed throughout the body, its distribution depending on:

- the perfusion of tissues by blood and
- the drug's plasma protein binding, lipid solubility and tissue binding.

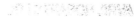

The brain is very well perfused and plasma protein binding, lipid solubility and tissue binding are therefore the major determinants of drug distribution within it.

Plasma protein binding

Drugs exist in the blood in two states, either bound to plasma proteins or unbound and free. The plasma proteins that bind drugs include albumin, globulins, lipoproteins and glycoproteins. Blood cells also bind drugs. Reduced albumin concentration or competition by another drug for binding sites may cause significant changes in plasma protein binding of a drug.

Plasma protein binding is extensive for most psychotropic drugs but only unbound drug is free to cross the blood–brain barrier (BBB), enter the brain and have an effect at a target neuroreceptor or enzyme. All psychotropic drugs are very lipid soluble and readily cross the BBB. Drugs that are very lipid soluble also pass rapidly into adipose tissue and they may continue to be released from these stores for weeks or even months after treatment with the drug has ceased.

Apparent volume of distribution

Plasma protein binding also influences the distribution of a drug in the body. The term 'apparent volume of distribution' is used to describe the volume of fluid required to contain the total amount of a drug in the body at the same concentration as in plasma. Thus if 100 mg of a drug is administered and all of it remains in the blood its apparent volume of distribution is equal to the volume of blood in the body or approximately 5 litres. However, if only 1 mg of the drug remains in the blood while 99 mg enters other tissues, the apparent volume of distribution will be 100 times the volume of blood in the body or approximately 500 litres.

Most psychotropic drugs bind extensively to plasma proteins and have a small apparent volume of distribution. Amfetamine, however, binds extensively to tissues and has an apparent volume of distribution that is greater than the volume of the body.

Metabolism

The metabolism of drugs generally occurs in two phases as follows:

- Phase I metabolism or biotransformation involves a chemical change to the drug by oxidation, hydrolysis or reduction. Ethanol undergoes oxidation to acetaldehyde, for example (see Fig. 14.1)
- Phase II metabolism or conjugation involves the addition of a further chemical group, for example by glucuronidation or methylation, in order

to produce a compound that is more water soluble and therefore more readily excreted by the kidneys.

Drugs are usually inactivated when they are metabolised. However, most psychotropic drugs have active metabolites and some of these are as active as the parent compound. Thus norfluoxetine and nortriptyline have AD activity equivalent to their parent compounds, fluoxetine and amitriptyline. Other drugs, referred to as 'prodrugs', are administered intentionally as inactive compounds in the knowledge that metabolism will activate them. For example, dopamine (DA), an effective treatment for Parkinson's disease, does not cross the BBB. However, L-dopa crosses it easily and is readily converted to DA in the brain. It is obvious, but perhaps nonetheless worth stating, that lithium, an element, cannot be metabolised.

Despite the fact that most psychotropic drugs are metabolised in the liver there are generally no restrictions on their use in patients with mild to moderate liver disease. Lithium, disulfiram and donepezil are safe in hepatic disease but

- phenothiazines are particularly hepatotoxic and should be avoided
- lofepramine and monoamine oxidase inhibitor AD drugs should be avoided
- sodium valproate is hepatotoxic and should be avoided
- the metabolism of benzodiazepine (BZD) drugs is impaired and those with long $T_{1/2}$ should be avoided and
- the dose of some atypical AP drugs (risperidone, sertindole) and some 5HT reuptake inhibitor AD drugs should be reduced.

Cytochrome P450 oxidase enzymes

Most psychotropic drugs are metabolised in the liver by cytochrome P-450 (CYP) oxidative enzymes. The CYP2D6 enzyme is probably the most important of these from a psychopharmacological perspective but CYP1A2, CYP2C9, CYP2C19, CYP2D6, CYP2E1 and CYP3A4 enzymes are also significant. In fact these six enzymes are responsible for over 90% of all drug oxidation in humans.

Variation in the genes coding for CYP2D6 enzymes may produce individuals who metabolise drugs either poorly (poor metabolisers or PMs) or extensively (extensive metabolisers or EMs). Between 5–10% of Caucasians are PMs, in contrast to approximately 2% of Asians. PMs are at increased risk of adverse effects from drugs metabolised by CYP2D6 while EMs may not respond at standard doses.

Drugs may increase or reduce the metabolism of other drugs by CYP (and other) enzyme systems as follows:

- An inducer is a drug that speeds up the metabolism of another drug either by inducing the activity of a CYP or other enzyme or by competing for enzymatic binding sites. This can be clinically significant. Carbamazepine and phenytoin, for example, induce the metabolism of ethinyloestradiol necessitating a 50 microgram dose for contraception rather than the usual 30–35 microgram dose (see Chapters 6 and 12).
- An inhibitor is a drug that slows down the metabolism of another drug by inhibiting a CYP enzyme. Fluoxetine, for example, inhibits CYP2D6 and slows down the metabolism of desimipramine.
- Fluvoxamine is somewhat unique in that it potently inhibits CYP1A2. Concomitant administration of fluvoxamine and either haloperidol or clozapine, both of which are metabolised by CYP1A2, may significantly increase their $T_{1/2}$ and plasma levels.

Elimination

Psychotropic drugs are generally eliminated from the body by renal excretion which depends on their metabolites being water soluble. Paraldehyde is exceptional in that it is excreted via the lungs. Renal excretion is the sum of three processes occurring simultaneously namely glomerular filtration (the most important), tubular secretion and tubular reabsorption.

The rate of elimination of a drug is usually proportional to its plasma concentration, a phenomenon referred to as first-order elimination kinetics. Some drugs are subject to zero-order elimination kinetics in which the elimination mechanisms rapidly become saturated so that elimination proceeds thereafter at a constant rate and is not proportional to the drug's plasma concentration. Alcohol becomes subject to zero-order kinetics once its plasma concentration reaches 10 mg per 100 ml, following which it is eliminated at a rate of approximately one unit per hour.

Despite the fact that psychotropic drugs are generally eliminated by renal excretion, there are generally no restrictions on the use of such drugs in patients with mild to moderate renal impairment. However:

- chloral hydrate, lithium and acamprosate should be avoided in patients with moderate renal impairment and
- clozapine is contraindicated in severe renal impairment.

Pharmacodynamics

Pharmacodynamics is the study of the beneficial and harmful effects of a drug on the body and of the mechanism of action of these effects.

Each class of psychotropic drug has its own pharmacodynamic properties which are described in the appropriate chapters of this book. In general however, psychotropic drugs may be regarded as having the following short-term and long-term pharmacodynamic effects.

Short-term pharmacodynamic effects

The principal mechanisms by which psychotropic drugs produce their pharmacodynamic effects in the short term include:

- promoting neurotransmitter release from the presynaptic membrane
- acting as agonists, antagonists or partial agonists at neuroreceptors
- allosteric modulation
- inhibiting neurotransmitter reuptake transporter proteins
- inhibiting catabolic enzymes and
- modifying second messenger systems.

Promotion of neurotransmitter release

Amfetamine is the best known example of a drug which produces its effect by promoting the release of neurotransmitter, in this case dopamine, from the presynaptic membrane into the synapse.

Some AD drugs, for example mirtazapine, also promote release of NA and serotonin (5HT) into the synapse. In this case, however, the mechanism of action is the prevention of negative feedback by synaptic NA and 5HT at presynaptic $NA_{\alpha2}$ and $5HT_{2A, 2C \& 3}$ autoreceptors (see Chapters 2 and 9).

Agonists, antagonists and partial agonists

A number of drugs produce their pharmacological effects by direct action at receptors where they may act as:

- agonists which bind to receptors and produce a response, for example morphine at the μ opioid receptor
- antagonists which bind to receptors and prevent a response by occupying the receptor and preventing an agonist binding to it. Naloxone, for example, will reverse respiratory depression and coma caused by opiates by displacing them from the μ opioid receptor. Rimonabant, a selective CB_1 receptor antagonist, has been marketed for the treatment of obesity and has also shown efficacy in smoking cessation (see Chapter 2)
- partial agonists bind to receptors and produce a submaximal response. Partial agonists may act like antagonists by blocking receptors and

preventing agonists from producing a response. Buprenorphine, for example, is a partial agonist at the μ opioid receptor that will prevent the pharmacological effects of opiates (see Chapter 14).

Allosteric modulation

BZD drugs are agonists at the $GABA_A$ receptor where they have an indirect rather than a direct effect in that they enhance the effect of GABA, the natural ligand and permit a greater influx of chloride ions than is possible through binding of GABA alone. This is an example of allosteric modulation (see Chapters 2 and 11).

Inhibition of neurotransmitter reuptake

Selective serotonin reuptake inhibitor AD drugs increase synaptic concentrations of 5HT by selectively inhibiting its reuptake via the 5HT transporter protein from the synapse to the presynaptic neurone. Serotonin and noradrenaline (norepinephrine) reuptake inhibitor AD drugs (and also some older AD drugs) inhibit the reuptake of both 5HT and NA via their transporter proteins (see Chapter 9).

Atomoxetine is a highly selective inhibitor of the NA reuptake transporter protein that is an effective treatment for attention deficit hyperactivity disorder (see Chapter 7).

Inhibition of catabolic enzymes

Monoamine oxidase inhibitors increase synaptic concentrations of noradrenaline (norepinephrine), 5HT and dopamine by irreversibly inhibiting MAO in the mitochondria of the terminal axon fibres and thus preventing their catabolism (see Chapters 2 and 9).

The antiepileptic drug vigabatrin similarly increases synaptic concentrations of gamma-amino butyric acid (GABA), the main inhibitory neurotransmitter in the brain, by inhibiting its catabolic enzyme GABA transaminase (see Chapter 12).

Anticholinesterase inhibitors for the treatment of dementia also utilise this mechanism of action (see Chapter 16) as do phospho-diesterase Type 5 inhibitors such as sildenafil which are effective treatments for erectile impotence (see Chapter 13).

Second messenger systems

Some psychotropic drugs may have a direct effect on second messengers. Lithium, for example, is thought to exert its effects by inhibiting the metabolism of phosphatidylinositol (see Chapter 10).

Caffeine similarly inhibits the metabolism of cyclic adenosine 3,5-monophosphate or cAMP.

Long-term pharmacodynamic effects

Long-term treatment with psychotropic drugs induces adaptive responses in the brain which may be beneficial or harmful. The most important of these responses include upregulation and down-regulation in numbers or sensitivity of neuroreceptors.

Neuroreceptor upregulation

One possible explanation for the delayed response to AD drugs is that increased concentrations of synaptic NA and 5HT induce increased numbers of postsynaptic neuroreceptors and this takes some weeks to occur.

It has also been suggested that long-term blockade of DA receptors by typical antipsychotic drugs may lead to a compensatory increase in their sensitivity which in turn causes tardive dyskinesia (Marsden and Jenner, 1980).

Neuroreceptor downregulation

A possible explanation of the tolerance and the discontinuation and withdrawal syndromes associated with alcohol, drugs of misuse and some prescribed psychotropic drugs is that downregulation in numbers or sensitivity of receptors induced by long-term use of a drug leads to inadequate neurotransmission when the drug is withdrawn. Thus, for example, long-term use of BZD drugs may lead to reduced numbers and sensitivity of GABA receptors such that stopping BZD treatment is associated with inadequate GABA-ergic neurotransmission and the typical symptoms of the BZD withdrawal syndrome (see Chapter 11) (Petursson and Lader, 1981).

Stereoisomerism

Stereoisomerism occurs when molecules with the same order of attachment of atoms have different three-dimensional structures because one atom, referred to as the chiral atom or centre and usually carbon, allows the atoms or side groups attached to it to have different orientations within the molecule (Pang, 1989). D-glucose and L-glucose are well-recognised examples of stereoisomers (D and L in these examples indicate that the molecules rotate polarised light to the right and left respectively).

A more precise description of stereoisomers is allowed by the R and S system which describes the spatial arrangement of atoms around the chiral centre of the molecule, for example the R-fluoxetine and S-fluoxetine stereoisomers or enantiomers.

Most psychotropic drugs are organic compounds that exhibit stereoisomerism and most are marketed as racemic mixtures of both enantiomers. Citalopram is unusual in that it is marketed both as a racemic mixture, citalopram, and as the pure S-citalopram enantiomer, escitalopram (see Chapter 9).

Enantiomers may differ significantly from each other in their pharmacokinetic, pharmacodynamic, therapeutic and safety profiles. Thus for example:

- S-warfarin and R-warfarin have $T_{1/2}$ of 30 and 50 hours respectively
- S-citalopram is 100 times more potent as an inhibitor of the 5HT transporter protein than R-citalopram and
- while R-thalidomide was a reasonably effective and safe hypnotic drug, S-thalidomide caused the well-known teratogenic adverse effect, phocomelia.

References and further reading

Electronic Medicines Compendium available online at http://emc.medicines.org.uk/ (accessed May 2005).

Marsden CD, Jenner P (1980) The pathophysiology of extrapyramidal side-effects of neuroleptic drugs. Psychological Medicine 10(1):55–72.

Pang Y (1989) Stereoisomerism in drug molecules. Australian Prescriber 12(1):19–25.

Petursson H, Lader MH (1981) Withdrawal from long term benzodiazepine treatment. British Medical Journal 283: 643–645.

Stahl SM (2000) Principles of chemical neurotransmission. In: Essential Psychopharmacology – Neuroscientific Basis and Practical Applications (2nd Edition). Cambridge, Cambridge University Press, pp. 199–243.

Wright P (2004) Psychopharmacology. In: Core Psychiatry (Eds Wright P, Phelan M and Stern J) (2nd Edition). London, Elsevier Saunders, pp. 579–609.

5

Invention and development of psychotropic drugs

Introduction

Pharmaceutical companies wishing to market a new prescription psychotropic drug for clinical use must satisfy the requirements of the regulatory authorities responsible for the country or region in which they wish the license to apply as to the drugs quality, safety and efficacy. Therefore following their invention, all such drugs must progress through stringent programmes of preclinical and clinical development before they are evaluated and approved for clinical use. This chapter provides a brief description of the regulatory approval process, drug invention and preclinical development and a more detailed account of clinical development and pharmacovigilance.

The regulatory approval process

The regulatory authority responsible for the member states of the European Union (EU) is the European Medicines Evaluation Agency (EMEA). The Food and Drug Administration (FDA) is the responsible regulatory authority for the United States. Similar organisations exist in other countries.

In addition to the EMEA, each of the 25 member states of the European Union has its own national regulatory agency, for example the Medicines and Healthcare products Regulatory Agency (MHRA) in the UK.

In addition to their role in licensing drugs the EMEA and national regulatory agencies play a vital role in monitoring the safety of drugs once approved and are empowered to take action in the event of concerns about safety (see below).

European Medicines Evaluation Agency

The EMEA was founded in 1995 and is responsible for protecting and promoting health by evaluating, approving and monitoring medicines for human and veterinary use. It has approved the marketing of more than 250 drugs to date.

Four committees exist within the EMEA that are responsible for evaluating and approving drugs for human use (Committee for Medicinal Products for Human Use or CHMP), drugs for veterinary use, orphan medicines and herbal medicines. The CHMP is composed of one member nominated by each of the national regulatory agencies of the member states of the EU, five further members with specific areas of expertise and a non-voting member from each of Norway, Iceland and Liechtenstein. In addition to the expertise of its members, the CHMP retains a panel of over 3000 experts and can obtain advice from the appropriate members of this panel when necessary.

The EMEA provides for the approval of drugs through a centralised procedure. This is compulsory for biotechnology products and for drugs for the treatment of AIDS, diabetes mellitus, cancer or neurodegenerative diseases. Other products may be approved through either this centralised procedure or through a mutual recognition procedure.

Centralised procedure

A pharmaceutical company wishing to license a drug via this procedure submits a single marketing authorisation application to the EMEA. This is evaluated by the national regulatory agency of one of the EU member states assisted by a second member state – the rapporteur and co-rapporteur member states respectively – on behalf of the CHMP. The CHMP reviews the member states' evaluation and adopts a positive opinion if satisfied about the drug's quality, safety and efficacy and convinced that it has a favourable benefit/risk profile. This positive opinion is subsequently converted into a marketing authorisation by the European Commission. A marketing authorisation permits the pharmaceutical company to market the drug in all 25 member states of the EU.

Mutual recognition procedure

A pharmaceutical company wishing to license a drug via this procedure submits a marketing authorisation application to one member state rather than to the EMEA. This is evaluated by the national regulatory agency of that state, thereafter referred to as the reference member state (RMS). The RMS adopts a positive opinion if satisfied about the drug's quality, safety and efficacy and convinced that it has a favourable benefit/risk profile. An application may then be submitted to other member states (the concerned member states or CMSs) who may subsequently accept or reject the opinion of the RMS. Rejection by a CMS leads to further discussion between the CMS(s) and the RMS and between the RMS and the pharmaceutical company who may be required to undertake further analyses or to perform further clinical trials. The application is referred to the CHMP if the RMS and CMSs cannot reach agreement. A marketing authorisation approved through the mutual recognition procedure permits the pharmaceutical company to market the drug in the RMS and CMSs and, ultimately, in all EU member states to whom the company makes an application.

Requirements for marketing authorisation approval

Irrespective of the approval procedure chosen, there are core requirements that all drugs submitted for marketing authorization approval must meet. In addition there are drug and/or disease-specific requirements that must be fulfilled. Thus for all drugs:

- adequate quality must be demonstrated – for example, the manufacturing process must ensure that a 10 mg tablet contains exactly 10 mg of the drug and

- adequate safety must be demonstrated – for example, the drug must not exhibit significant teratogenicity or oncogenicity. Safety data must be collected over a treatment period that reflects the actual use of the drug. This may be a matter of some weeks with antibiotics but in the case of most psychotropic drugs which patients may take for several years, data must be collected over at least 12 months.

Examples of drug- and/or disease-specific requirements that must be fulfilled include the need to demonstrate that an antidepressant (AD) drug is more effective than placebo and at least as effective as an AD drug that is already marketed. In addition, it must be demonstrated that an AD drug is capable of preventing relapse (worsening of a current episode) and recurrence (the development of a new episode) of depression.

The EMEA's core and drug- and/or disease-specific requirements are documented in *Note for Guidance* documents which they publish for most diseases, for example *Note for Guidance on Clinical Investigation of Medicinal Products for the Treatment and Prevention of Bipolar Disorder* (2001). Pharmaceutical companies also obtain scientific advice from CHMP following the submission of briefing documents that outline their proposed clinical development of a drug.

Summary of Product Characteristics

A document referred to as the Summary of Product Characteristics (SPC) is prepared by pharmaceutical companies and modified and approved by the CHMP for every drug that receives a marketing authorisation approval from the EMEA. The SPC, often referred to colloquially as the license or label (hence the term 'off label' applied to the use of a drug in a manner not specified in its SPC or to treat a disease for which it is not approved), lists the diseases the drug may be prescribed to treat, provides advice on dosing and warns about adverse effects and interactions with other drugs. The SPCs for all drugs approved for use in the UK are available online at Electronic Medicines Compendium.

Drug invention

Drug invention depends on knowledge of the disease being targeted and/or knowledge of other drugs available to treat that disease. Serendipity also plays a significant role (see Chapter 2).

Chemists wishing to invent a new drug may base their initial molecular designs on an endogenous molecule known to be implicated in the pathophysiology of the disease being targeted. For example, given that dopamine (DA) has been implicated in schizophrenia, a chemist might attempt to design a molecule that is sufficiently similar to the DA molecule that it will bind to DA receptors but yet sufficiently different from DA that it will not activate these receptors.

Rational drug invention based on knowledge of the disease being targeted may be the ideal and indeed it is one of the hopes that underpins the Human Genome Project (see Chapter 2). However, it is difficult to accomplish in practice. This is especially true in the case of psychiatric diseases where pathophysiology is imperfectly under-stood. Many psychotropic drugs were therefore discovered by chance. However, their existence permits the invention of newer psychotropic drugs based on knowledge of the mechanisms of action or safety profiles of these older drugs. Thus the atypical antipsychotic (AP) drug olanzapine, invented in 1986, is the result of an effort to invent a molecule with the efficacy of clozapine, invented in 1958, but without its propensity to cause agranulocytosis (see Chapter 8).

Some of the techniques of drug invention have been discussed in Chapter 2 including combinatorial chemistry, high-throughput screening, pharmacoelectroencephalography and pharmacogenomics. Two further disciplines are making an increasing contribution to drug invention – pharmacoproteomics and biomarker science.

Pharmacoproteomics

Pharmacoproteomics may be defined as the study of the expression, modification and metabolism of proteins and of their interactions with each other and with genes. Much academic and pharmaceutical research is directed at determining the role in health and disease of the approximately 200,000 proteins in the human body in the hope that this will facilitate drug invention. It is likely that this hope will gradually be fulfilled given that over 500 of the drugs currently available have proteins, usually receptors or enzymes, as their target sites of action.

Biomarker science

Biomarkers were originally described in relation to cancers and were defined as substances in blood, other body fluids or tissues that indicated susceptibility to, the presence of and/or the severity of disease. Many biomarkers also provide a measure of response to treatment. Well-known examples of biomarkers include carcino-embryonic antigen or CEA in colorectal cancer and prostate specific antigen or PSA in prostatic cancer. Blood glucose in diabetes mellitus and erythrocyte sedimentation rate in connective tissue disease are also biomarkers although they are not usually referred to as such. Biomarkers are now divided into those that are directly involved in the pathophysiology of disease, for example blood glucose in diabetes mellitus, and those that are surrogate markers of disease, for example low-density lipoproteins in atherosclerosis. Advances in biomarker science may increase our knowledge of pathophysiology and aid drug invention and development. It is also likely that the evaluation of biomarkers will become a regulatory requirement for many diseases.

A drug's journey from its initial design on a chemist's computer screen to clinical use is uncertain, prolonged and expensive. Uncertain because only 1 in every 5000 to 10,000 of the drugs that are invented achieves regulatory approval. Prolonged because the performance of the preclinical and clinical trials required for regulatory approval may take 10–15 years. And expensive because the average cost of inventing, developing, licensing and marketing a drug now exceeds £500 million or approximately $1 billion.

Preclinical development

Only 250 out of every 5,000 drugs invented will enter the preclinical stage of development. The primary purpose of this stage is to determine a drug's safety before it is administered to humans. Preclinical development therefore includes:

- quality testing to establish the drug's purity and to determine its stability and shelf-life
- *in vitro* toxicological and pharmacodynamic testing in cultured cells and tissues and
- *in vivo* toxicological, pharmacokinetic and pharmacodynamic testing in a range of animals (rodents, non-rodents and primates) and
- behavioural psychopharmacology studies.

Behavioural psychopharmacology

Preclinical behavioural psychopharmacology is essentially the study of the effects of psychotropic drugs on the behaviour and cognition of animals. Behavioural psychopharmacologists undertake studies during the preclinical development of a psychotropic drug in order to determine:

- whether it has efficacy in animal models of the disease being targeted. It will be appreciated that while animal models of diabetes mellitus or renal failure are very reliable, animal models of psychiatric disease provide limited evidence of the drug efficacy. The forced swim test, for example, is used extensively as a screening test for AD drugs. It relies on the fact that rodents placed in a tank of water from which they cannot escape will discontinue energetic swimming and attempting to climb the walls of the tank after approximately 10 minutes on first exposure and after approximately 2 minutes on subsequent exposure. Effective AD drugs prolong energetic swimming and climbing activity, often in a dose-dependent manner;
- whether it induces dependency. Rodents can be induced to become dependent on alcohol and a range of drugs of misuse. Tests can then be designed to determine if these animals prefer the drug under development to alcohol or drugs of misuse; and
- whether it causes undesirable effects such as cognitive impairment or altered sleep architecture. A drug's propensity to cause cognitive impairment, for example, may be evaluated by training rodents to undertake complex tasks and then measuring their ability to do so following treatment with the drug under development.

Behavioural psychopharmacology studies are also undertaken during clinical development when the effects of psychotropic drugs on, for example, cognitive function, driving ability and sleep architecture are evaluated through cognitive testing and the use of driving simulators and sleep laboratories.

Clinical development

Only five out of every 250 drugs that enter the preclinical stage of development will progress to full-scale clinical development. The other 245 will be abandoned because of toxicity, for pharmacokinetic reasons (poor absorption for example, or very limited bioavailability because of extensive first pass metabolism and the absence of active metabolites), for pharmacodynamic reasons (the drug does not adequately bind to the targeted receptors for example) or for pharmaceutical reasons (it is impossible to ensure adequate quality of the drug or the manufacturing process cannot be economically or safely scaled up to industrial proportions).

Clinical development consists of clinical trials designed and performed by physicians employed by pharmaceutical companies in collaboration with physicians working in hospitals or primary care. Several pharmaceutical companies now list all the clinical trials they have performed or are performing on their websites (see, for example, the websites of GlaxoSmithKline and Eli Lilly and Company).

Clinical development is traditionally divided into Phases I, II, III and IV, each of which will now be briefly described.

Phase I clinical development

The clinical trials undertaken during Phase I development are designed to determine the safety and pharmacokinetics of the new drug, to evaluate drug–drug interactions and, when possible, to determine dose. Thus open-label, single, escalating and multiple-dose clinical trials are undertaken in small numbers (<100) of healthy volunteers. The majority of volunteers are male because the teratogenic potential of a drug has not yet been determined at this stage. Phase I trials take place in specialized, well-staffed and highly equipped research units that are either commercial enterprises or associated with large university hospitals.

Phase I trials generally extend over 1–2 years and typically take place at one or two research centres in one or two countries. Functional neuroimaging and pharmacoelectroencephalography are increasingly used during the Phase I development of psychotropic drugs (see Chapter 2).

Phase II clinical development

The clinical trials undertaken during Phase II development are designed to further evaluate safety (especially safety in multiple dosing and with prolonged treatment), pharmacokinetics and pharmacodynamics, and to determine appropriate dosages and dosing regimens. So called 'proof of concept' trials, in which the efficacy of the drug being developed in treating the disease being targeted is evaluated, are a vital component of Phase II clinical development. Thus open-label and double-blind, single, escalating and multiple-dose clinical trials are performed in relatively small numbers of patients (<500) suffering with the disease the new drug is intended to treat. Placebo controlled trials may also be undertaken.

Phase II trials generally extend over 2–4 years and take place at a small number of research centres in a few countries. As with Phase I development, functional neuroimaging and electroencephalography are increasingly used during the Phase II development of psychotropic drugs.

Phase III clinical development

The clinical trials undertaken during Phase III development are designed to provide statistical evidence that the drug being developed is more effective than placebo and at least as effective and safe as a comparator drug (a drug that has already been licensed to treat the disease being investigated). Phase III trials of psychotropic drugs usually involve large numbers of patients (2000 or more), both hospitalised and outpatient, who are randomised to double-blind treatment with the drug being developed (which may be administered in fixed or flexible doses), a comparator drug or placebo.

Most readers will be familiar with Phase III clinical trials because their results are usually reported in major medical or psychiatric journals. Readers of such reports should bear in mind that Phase III clinical trials are undertaken primarily in order to meet the needs of regulatory authorities and to obtain a marketing authorisation approval for the drug being developed. They are not undertaken for the primary purpose of answering questions about the treatment of patients. The requirements of the former are similar to, but nonetheless differ significantly from, those of the latter. The patients and treatments involved in clinical trials of psychotropic drugs therefore differ greatly from those involved in clinical practice in that:

- Only patients who meet stringent inclusion and exclusion criteria are enrolled in clinical trials whereas all patients who present to a clinician must be treated in clinical practice.
- An excess of male patients are enrolled in clinical trials.
- Operational diagnostic systems, typically the 4th edition of the *Diagnostic and Statistical Manual of the American Psychiatric Association* (2000), are employed in clinical trials whilst patients in clinical practice are diagnosed 'clinically'.

- Only patients who exhibit a relatively narrow range of symptom severity are enrolled in clinical trials. Thus a minimum score on a symptom scale, for example a Positive and Negative Syndrome Scale (Kay, Opler and Fizbein, 1987) score of $\geq$ 70 in the case of schizophrenia, is necessary to permit inclusion whilst the need to provide informed consent and cooperate with the requirements of the trial excludes patients with severe symptomatology.
- Patients subject to mental health legislation are generally excluded from clinical trials.
- Patients with comorbid diseases, either medical or psychiatric, are excluded from clinical trials both because the safety of the drug being investigated may not yet be known in patients with, for example, hepatic failure, and in order to ensure that any clinical change observed is caused exclusively by the drug under investigation.
- Patients who misuse illicit drugs are generally excluded from clinical trials in order to ensure that any clinical change observed is caused exclusively by the drug under investigation.
- The administration of concomitant medication is prohibited or carefully controlled in clinical trials in order to ensure that any clinical change observed is caused exclusively by the drug under investigation.
- The treatment, both drug and dosage, a patient receives in a clinical trial is directed by the trial protocol and is usually administered in a double-blind fashion.
- The frequency of clinical assessments and laboratory investigations and the close monitoring of compliance with treatment that are typical of clinical trials differs significantly from clinical practice.

Phase III trials generally extend over 5 years or more and take place at many research centres in many countries and often on several continents.

Phase IV clinical development

Phase IV clinical development occurs once a drug receives marketing authorisation approval from a regulatory authority. The clinical trials undertaken during Phase IV development are designed to investigate the efficacy and safety of the drug in:

- less stringently defined groups of the patients that it is approved to treat. For example an AP drug may be studied in patients with a clinical diagnosis of schizophrenia who misuse cannabis as distinct from patients with an operational diagnosis who do not

- less severely or more severely ill groups of the patients that it is licensed to treat. The need to provide informed consent and cooperate with the requirements of a clinical trial means that it is not possible, for example, to investigate a parenteral AP drug in the severely agitated patients it is designed to treat prior to approval (Wright et al, 2001). Once licensed, however, this drug may be administered legitimately to such patients and its effects observed.

Observational (or naturalistic) trials are frequently performed during Phase IV clinical development. Such trials seek to observe and record patients' symptoms, the treatment they receive, and the benefits and adverse effects of such treatment, in ordinary clinical practice. Data from observational trials are not suitable for making comparisons, especially efficacy comparisons, between drugs because prescriptions are not issued in a randomised, double-blind manner and, because many objective and subjective factors influence the drug a clinician prescribes for any individual patient.

Pharmacovigilance

Pharmacovigilance may be defined as the continuous monitoring of the safety of drugs after they receive marketing authorisation. Both the EMEA and national regulatory authorities such as the MHRA in the UK undertake this role and coordinate any action that may be necessary in relation to the safety and quality of a drug. Safety data are obtained from two sources, clinical trials and clinical practice.

Safety data from clinical trials

It will be evident from the discussion on Phase IV clinical development that clinical trials continue after a drug has received marketing authorisation. In addition to Phase IV trials, Phase I, II and III trials are also commonly undertaken after marketing authorisation has been obtained. Such trials are necessary if a pharmaceutical company wishes to license a drug for the treatment of further diseases (for example an AP drug licensed initially for the treatment of schizophrenia may subsequently be licensed for the treatment of acute mania) or if new formulations of a drug are developed (in the case of an AP drug for example, tablets or capsules may be licensed initially and subsequent trials undertaken with liquid, rapidly acting intra-muscular or depot intramuscular formulations). Safety data collected from such trials must be evaluated and reported by pharmaceutical companies to the EMEA and/or national regulatory authorities at regular intervals.

Safety data from clinical practice

Clinicians who prescribe drugs have a professional responsibility to report the adverse effects that their patients experience to national regulatory authorities and/or the manufacturer of the drug concerned. All adverse effects should be reported in the case of newly licensed drugs and severe adverse effects in the case of established drugs. Serious adverse events are defined as those which:

- cause or prolong hospitalisation
- cause significant disability or incapacity
- produce a congenital abnormality
- are life-threatening or
- are fatal.

Reports of adverse effects may be made in the UK via 'yellow cards' (included in the British National Formulary) submitted to the Committee on Safety of Medicines (CSM), an independent advisory committee to the MHRA, or via the CSM or MHRA websites. The CSM evaluate all reports received via 'yellow cards' and advise the MHRA on any appropriate action to take. The CSM also regularly send *Current Problems in Pharmacovigilance*, their drug safety bulletin, to all doctors, dentists, pharmacists and coroners in the UK. This alerts clinicians to problems with drugs and provides advice on safer prescribing. The bulletin is also available from the MHRA website.

Reports of adverse effects received directly by pharmaceutical companies from clinicians are investigated by such companies and further data collected. These data are evaluated and incorporated into the regular safety reports made by pharmaceutical companies to the EMEA and/or national regulatory authorities.

Regulatory authority actions in the event of safety concerns about a drug

It has been noted above that in addition to their role in licensing drugs the EMEA and national regulatory agencies play a vital role in monitoring the safety of licensed drugs and taking action in the event of concerns about safety. A range of such actions is available including:

- Addition of further advice and warnings to the drugs SPC and to its Patient Information Leaflet or PIL, the document included with every package of drugs.
- Issuance of a product safety announcement – this consists of a press release and an announcement on the EMEA or national regulatory

agency's website which provides further advice and warnings about the drug both to clinicians and to patients. Product safety announcements are invariably accompanied by changes to the drug's SPC.

- Issuance of a Dear Doctor (more correctly a Dear Healthcare Provider) Letter – the content of such letters is proposed by the pharmaceutical company concerned and modified and approved by the EMEA or national regulatory agency. Letters are sent to appropriate doctors, for example the specialists most likely to prescribe the drug, and to all general practitioners and all pharmacists. Dear Doctor Letters are usually posted on the EMEA or national regulatory agency websites. They are invariably accompanied by changes to the drug's SPC and PIL.

- Suspension of marketing authorisation – the effect of this action is that clinicians can no longer prescribe the drug and a pharmaceutical company cannot market it until further safety data are collected. Such data may lead to either reinstatement or withdrawal of the marketing authorisation.

- Withdrawal of marketing authorisation – the effect of this action is that clinicians can no longer prescribe the drug and a pharmaceutical company cannot market it. Transitional measures such as making the drug available on a named patient basis may be put in place to provide for patients already taking the drug and obtaining significant benefit without significant ill effect.

Which action is taken and the speed with which it is imposed will depend on the disease the drug is intended to treat, the adverse effects reported and the availability of alternative treatments. More severe adverse effects are clearly acceptable in the case of cytotoxic drugs intended to treat cancer, for example, than in the case of drugs intended to treat headache.

References and further reading

American Psychiatric Association (2000) 4th Edition of the Diagnostic and Statistical Manual (Text Revision). Washington, American Psychiatric Association.

Committee on Safety of Medicines. Available online at http://medicines.mhra.gov.uk/aboutagency/regframework/csm/csmhome.htm (accessed May 2005).

Electronic Medicines Compendium. Available online at http://www.emc.medicines.org.uk (accessed September 2004 through May 2005).

Eli Lilly and Company. Available online at http://www.lillytrials.com (accessed May 2005).

European Medicines Evaluation Agency. Available online at http://www.emea.eu.int/ (accessed May 2005).

Food and Drug Administration. Available online at http://www.fda.gov/default.htm (accessed May 2005).

GlaxoSmithKline. Available online at http://ctr.gsk.co.uk (accessed May 2005).

Kay SR, Opler LA, Fizbein A (1987) The Positive and Negative Syndrome Scale (PANSS) for schizophrenia. Schizophrenia Bulletin 13:261–276.

Medicines and Healthcare products Regulatory Agency. Available online at http://www.mhra.gov.uk/ (accessed May 2005).

Note for Guidance on Clinical Investigation of Medicinal Products for the Treatment and Prevention of Bipolar Disorder (2001) Available online at http://www.emea.eu.int/pdfs/human/ewp/056798en.pdf (accessed May 2005).

Wright P, Birkett M, David S, et al (2001) Double blind, placebo controlled comparison of intramuscular olanzapine and intramuscular haloperidol in the treatment of acute agitation in schizophrenia. American Journal of Psychiatry 158: 1149–1151.

Part II
Clinical Psychopharmacology

6

Introduction to clinical psychopharmacology

Introduction

The syllabus for the Part I and Part II membership examinations of the Royal College of Psychiatrists requires a trainee psychiatrist to have:

- an appreciation of the relevance of psychopharmacology to the practice of psychiatry
- an understanding of personal and social factors that influence the willingness of patients to take medication
- an understanding of genetic and personal factors that influence an individual patient's response to medication, both beneficial and harmful
- knowledge of the main classes of psychotropic drugs including their postulated mechanisms of action, the influence of such mechanisms on our understanding of the pathophysiology of psychiatric illness and the principal efficacy and safety differences between the members of the main classes of psychotropic drugs
- knowledge of the adverse effects of psychotropic drugs and of their interactions with other psychotropic and non-psychotropic drugs
- an understanding of the placebo effect and
- an understanding of functional neuroimaging and its contribution to the development of psychotropic drugs.

Part II of this book consists of this chapter, which discusses the general principles of clinical psychopharmacology, the placebo effect and the drug treatment of special populations of patients, and a further

11 chapters that provide accounts of each of the main classes of psychotropic drugs and of their use in the treatment of specific groups of patients or specific psychiatric syndromes. These chapters focus on psychotropic drugs available in the UK. Such drugs are almost always available in other countries. In contrast, however, drugs available in other countries may not be available in the UK. The final chapter in this section provides an account of the psychopharmacology of electroconvulsive therapy.

The advice on treatment contained in this and the following chapters refers only to the use of psychotropic drugs. A textbook of psychiatry should be consulted for a description of the comprehensive treatment – educational, psychological, social and physical as well as psychopharmacological – of patients with psychiatric disorders.

General principles of clinical psychopharmacology

A number of general principles apply to the practice of clinical psycho-pharmacology. Most are obvious and derive from common sense. These bear repeating. A few are technical. These require explanation.

Clinical knowledge and clinical experience are the foundations upon which the effective and safe practice of clinical psycho-pharmacology is founded.

Clinical knowledge

Textbooks such as this one provide a useful service to psychiatrists in that they present up-to-date knowledge in summary format in a single volume. However, our knowledge of drugs is advancing constantly and the most up-to-date sources of information available should be consulted regularly, and particularly before prescribing a recently licensed drug. In the UK these sources include:

1. The Summary of Product Characteristics (SPC) (see Chapter 5), available from the manufacturer of a drug and also available online through the Electronic Medicines Compendium (http://www.emc.medicines.org.uk).
2. The current British National Formulary (BNF), also available online (www.bnf.org).
3. The guidance available from the National Institute of Clinical Excellence (NICE), available online (www.nice.org.uk).
4. The guidance available from the Committee on Safety of Medicines (CSM), available online (http://medicines.mhra.gov.uk/aboutagency/regframework/csm/csmhome.htm).

5. The guidance available from the Royal College of Psychiatrists, available online (www.rcpsych.ac.uk/).

Clinical experience

Experience in clinical psychopharmacology should focus initially on depth rather than breadth. Thus psychiatrists should generally adhere to the following 'rules':

- **Always consider non-drug treatment before prescribing** – advice on lifestyle or psychological treatment may be more appropriate than medication. This is particularly the case in patients who complain of 'stress' or of sleep disturbance/insomnia.
- **Limit prescribing to two or three drugs from each of the main classes of psychotropic drugs** – this allows depth of experience with these drugs to be developed, both in significant numbers of patients and over significant durations of treatment. Such experience helps greatly when evaluating the efficacy and safety of drugs and when explaining their benefits and risks to patients.
- **Limit prescribing to established rather than recently licensed drugs** – this is because personal and general knowledge and experience are more extensive for the former. For example it is generally better to prescribe an established antidepressant (AD) drug such as fluoxetine, citalopram or venlafaxine rather than a more recently licensed AD drug. The latter should be reserved, at least initially, for patients who have not benefited from established drugs or who may derive significant advantage from some specific efficacy or safety characteristic of the new drug.
- **Aim for monotherapy** – this frequently cited goal should generally be achievable when treating patients suffering from an anxiety disorder or from depression. However, a proportion of such patients will require medications in addition to AD drugs, for example an anxiolytic or hypnotic drug prescribed for a few weeks. Monotherapy is less often possible when treating patients with schizophrenia or bipolar disorder. The former require antipsychotic (AP) drugs but also frequently benefit from AD, anxiolytic or hypnotic drugs. The latter need a mood stabilising drug such as lithium but may also require AP, AD, anxiolytic or hypnotic drugs. It therefore seems reasonable to advise that a psychiatrist should aim for monotherapy while recognising that it is not appropriate for every patient. Certainly no patient should be denied access to a drug from which they may gain benefit because of rigid adherence to the principle of monotherapy.
- **Prescribe only one drug from any class of psychotropic drugs at a time** – there is generally no advantage, for example, to prescribing two or more selective serotonin reuptake inhibitor (SSRI) AD drugs.

- **Prescribe within your knowledge and experience** – prescribing that differs significantly from mainstream clinical practice is the exception rather than the rule, even among experienced experts at tertiary referral centres. And while occasional depressed patients, for example, respond only to combination treatment with three AD drugs from three different classes of AD, such treatment regimens should only be prescribed following consultation with experienced colleagues when standard regimens have proven ineffective, and with appropriate monitoring.

- **Be aware of drug interactions** – all other drugs that a patient is taking must be considered carefully before a psychotropic drug is prescribed. This advice is especially important when treating substance misusing patients (who may be taking some or all of 'over the counter' medications, prescribed drugs, illegally obtained prescription drugs and 'street' drugs) and when prescribing for women and elderly patients (see below).

- **Change only one drug or dose at a time** – it is almost inevitable that either the drug itself or its dosage will need to be changed at some point. Only one change should be made at a time because this allows the effectiveness of that change to be evaluated. If two or more changes are made it is impossible to determine which is responsible for any beneficial or harmful outcome.

- **Aim for patient-friendly treatment regimens** – most psychotropic drugs have a prolonged duration of effect and may be prescribed once daily and taken at any time of the day. Patients are far more likely to take one tablet once daily at a time that suits them rather than different numbers of tablets at varying intervals during the day.

- **Consider the various formulations of drugs that are available** – available formulations include hard tablets, capsules, orally disintegrating tablets and liquid. Many patients who are not prepared to take hard tablets or capsules will agree to take orally disintegrating tablets or liquid.

- **Wait** – psychotropic drugs take time to achieve their maximum effect. Warn patients about this and resist the temptation (and the pressure from others) to change treatment too soon.

Advising patients about psychotropic drugs

Historically, psychiatrists have told patients very little about the psychotropic drugs prescribed for them. More recently, educating patients about their drugs has become one of a psychiatrist's key responsibilities. This change has been stimulated by a realisation that only patients who are knowledgeable about the benefits and risks of the drugs they take:

- may provide informed consent to that treatment
- are likely to take medication as prescribed and
- are able to collaborate in a therapeutic alliance in which the psychiatrist explains the benefits and risks of drugs, prescribes them and monitors their effect, while the patient takes such drugs as instructed and reports beneficial and harmful experiences to the psychiatrist.

A further stimulus to this change has been patients' own increasing knowledge about drugs, facilitated by the internet and by the inclusion of a detailed Product Information Leaflet (PIL) written in non-technical language in every packet of drugs.

Before any psychotropic drug is prescribed, every patient should be advised about:

- the drug's anticipated benefits
- its commonly experienced adverse effects
- the period of time over which beneficial and adverse effects may occur (the efficacy of AD drugs takes some weeks to manifest for example, while some AD drugs cause abdominal cramps after a few days and sexual dysfunction in the longer term in a significant proportion of patients)
- the duration of treatment that is necessary (patients being prescribed AD drugs for the first time will not be aware that treatment may need to continue for a year or longer and patients being treated for schizophrenia or bipolar disorder will not anticipate the need for lifelong treatment) and
- the importance of not discontinuing treatment without advice because of the risk of relapse and of discontinuation syndrome (for example in the case of many AD drugs).

Initial advice to patients will necessarily be verbal. This should be supplemented by written information, either in the form of a letter to the patient or as a leaflet such as those available from the Royal College of Psychiatrists or, preferably, both. Patients should also be encouraged to obtain further information about their drugs from the internet and from PILs and advised to write down questions they wish to ask at subsequent consultations.

Educating patients is particularly important when a psychotropic drug is prescribed to treat a disease for which it is not licensed. Such prescribing is appropriate when documented in textbooks or other sources such as those listed at the beginning of this chapter, and when supported by standard clinical practice. For example it is recognised that a low dose of risperidone may be beneficial if prescribed in combination with an AD drug for a patient with obsessive compulsive disorder. It goes without saying that such a patient, unless forewarned, will be surprised to read the risperidone PIL and find that it is indicated, not for obsessive compulsive disorder, but for schizophrenia.

Similarly, it is reasonable to prescribe a drug above its maximum licensed dose if a patient has experienced partial efficacy at this dose and has not experienced troublesome adverse effects. The rationale behind such prescribing should be discussed carefully with the patient and documented in the medical records and the patient's clinical status should be carefully monitored.

The placebo effect

The placebo effect refers to the fact that a proportion of patients suffering from any given disease will experience a reduction in their symptoms if administered an inactive drug. Patients may also experience adverse effects when treated with such a drug (sometimes called the nocebo effect).

Possible explanations for the placebo effect include:

- Psychological mechanisms – the efficacy of psychological treatments such as cognitive therapy has been proven and it may be that the neurobiological mechanisms that underpin these treatments are also responsible for the placebo effect (Benedetti and Amanzio, 1997). The patient's beliefs and hopes and the clinician's expectations may play a role in this.

- Natural history of the disease – the symptoms of disease fluctuate and patients eventually recover from many diseases. It may be that the placebo effect is no more than a measure of the proportion of patients with any disease who were due to recover as the disease ran its natural course.

- Non-specific treatments – patients who receive placebos do not remain untreated. In the context of a clinical trial for example, such patients will receive standard medical care – a sympathetic and helpful relationship with a physician, assessment, investigation, validation of their symptoms and experiences, education, monitoring – with the exception of treatment with an active drug. Most psychiatrists, and indeed most physicians, would accept that such non-specific treatment is highly beneficial to a considerable proportion of patients.

In general, the placebo response is:
- evident much earlier than the usual response to a drug. For example response to AD drugs is usually only evident after some weeks whereas the placebo response in depressed patients may occur within days

- more evident in patients with anxiety disorders and depression and less evident in those with schizophrenia and bipolar disorder and
- more evident in patients with acute disorders and less evident in those with chronic disorders.

Clinical trials

It is usually necessary to demonstrate that a new psychotropic drug is more effective than placebo and at least as effective as a similar drug that is already marketed before it is approved for clinical use (see Chapter 5).

Placebo response rates in clinical trials involving patients with depression may be as high as 60% (Hróbjartsson and Götzsche, 2001). It will be appreciated that there are few active AD drugs that could hope to exceed this to a statistically significant extent. And even in clinical trials involving patients with schizophrenia who are agitated, placebo response rates of 33% have been reported (Wright et al, 2001).

Controlling for placebo response is therefore a vital element of the design of clinical trials. This may be achieved to some extent by a placebo run in period of perhaps two weeks' duration during which all patients in the trial are treated with placebo and following which only those who do not respond to placebo are randomised to double-blind treatment, i.e. those who respond are removed from the trial. It may also be achieved by recruiting 'enriched patient samples' who have more severe and/or more chronic disease and are therefore less likely to respond to placebo.

Future clinical trials may include not only groups of patients randomised to the drug being investigated, to an active comparator and to placebo, but also to an 'active placebo' and to 'no treatment'. An active placebo is a drug that would mimic the adverse effects of the drug being investigated but have none of that drug's potential efficacy. Thus in a clinical trial of an AP drug a sedative might be administered to mimic any sedating properties of the AP drug. The purpose of an active placebo is to prevent inadvertent unblinding of clinicians or patients caused by adverse effects. The purpose of a 'no treatment' arm is to exclude non-specific treatment effects.

Special populations of patients

The treatment of children, women and elderly patients with psychotropic drugs merits special attention because human pharmacokinetics change with age and because some drugs pose a risk before and during pregnancy and in the neonate. Care must also be exercised when prescribing psychotropic drugs for motorists or individuals who operate machinery.

Children

The detailed treatment of children with psychiatric disorders is discussed in Chapter 7. Children require great care when treating them with psychotropic drugs because:

- they generally absorb, metabolise and eliminate drugs more rapidly than adults
- formulations may not be available to allow precise dosing based upon body weight and
- drugs are not extensively tested in children during clinical development. Thus most psychotropic drugs used to treat children are prescribed 'off label' in that they are not specifically licensed for use in children.

There are few psychotropic drugs that are specifically indicated for the treatment of psychiatric disorder in children. Equally, there are few that are specifically contraindicated (but see Chapter 9 for CSM advice on the use of SSRI AD drugs for the treatment of major depressive disorder in individuals under 18 years of age. It should be noted that the use of psychotropic drugs in children is an area of very active interest to the CSM who have recently issued advice on a number of occasions). A current reference such as the BNF and the appropriate SPC should therefore be consulted before prescribing any psychotropic drug for patients under 18 years of age.

Women

Women are largely excluded from clinical trials of new drugs because the potential teratogenic and reproductive effects of such drugs are then unknown. Yet women receive twice as many prescriptions for psychotropic drugs as men. The treatment of female patients with such drugs during their reproductive years therefore requires particular care.

Oral contraceptive pill

Psychotropic drugs that induce hepatic enzymes and increase the metabolism of both the combined and progesterone only oral contraceptives include carbamazepine, phenytoin, modafinil, phenobarbital and primidone. Women taking such drugs should either use an alternative method of contraception or take an oral contraceptive that provides 50 micrograms of ethinyloestradiol per day (see Chapter 12).

Reproductive function

Psychoactive drugs should be avoided in women who are planning to become pregnant or who are already pregnant. However, this is not always possible and when a decision is taken to commence or continue a psychoactive drug during pregnancy because the potential benefits outweigh the potential risks, the following guidelines should be applied:

- Ensure that women who are taking antiepileptic drugs as mood stabilisers or for epilepsy take appropriate doses of folate supplements both before conception and during pregnancy in order to reduce the risk of neural tube defects (such advice is now applicable to all women contemplating pregnancy).
- If possible, avoid treatment during the first trimester when the risk of teratogenicity is greatest.
- Use the lowest effective dose possible.
- Use established rather than recently introduced drugs because more information on their use during pregnancy is available.
- Consult the manufacturer of a drug for up-to-date information on its use in pregnancy.

Drugs of choice during pregnancy include carbamazepine and fluoxetine. Acamprosate, antiepileptic drugs other than carbamazepine, benzodiazepines, tricyclic AD drugs, lithium and quetiapine should be avoided.

Most psychotropic drugs are secreted in breast milk and although concentrations may be low, breast-feeding infants are at risk of the same adverse effects as adults taking such drugs. Guidelines similar to those applied to pregnant women should therefore be applied to women who are breast feeding. Breast-feeding women may take AD drugs but should avoid acamprosate, lithium, risperidone (risk of dystonia), clozapine (risk of agranulocytosis) and quetiapine.

Hyperprolactinaemia

Typical AP drugs such as haloperidol frequently cause hyper-prolactinaemia which in turn causes hypo-oestrogenaemia, anovulation and amenorrhoea. Sexually active women taking such drugs are therefore relatively unlikely to become pregnant. Women switched from typical AP drugs to atypical AP drugs that do not cause hyper-prolactinaemia (the so-called prolactin-sparing atypical AP drugs such as aripiprazole, clozapine and olanzapine) should be advised about the return of menstruation and the risk of pregnancy.

Hyperprolactinaemia caused by typical AP drugs may cause hypo-oestrogenaemia and increase the risk of osteoporosis. Prolactin-sparing atypical AP drugs may therefore be particularly appropriate when treating female patients.

Elderly patients

Elderly patients experience twice as many adverse effects as younger patients because:

* drug absorption, metabolism and elimination decrease with age
* such patients frequently suffer from significant systemic diseases and
* drug interactions are more likely because such patients may require simultaneous treatment with several drugs.

Psychotropic drugs should be commenced at the lowest possible dose in elderly patients, the dose being increased slowly thereafter while vigilance is maintained for adverse effects. This practice is well summarised in the adage 'start low and go slow'. Confusion is a frequent adverse effect of such drugs in elderly patients and drug-induced postural hypotension or sedation may lead to falls that result in hip fractures and fatalities.

Motorists

Many psychotropic drugs cause impaired attention, drowsiness and sedation, particularly when treatment is initially commenced or dosage is increased. Patients who drive or who operate machinery should be warned of these effects and advised of the synergistic effects of such drugs with each other and with alcohol. They should be specifically warned that it is illegal to drive while driving ability is impaired by drugs, even if these drugs are prescribed.

References and further reading

Benedetti F, Amanzio M (1997) The neurobiology of placebo analgesia: from endogenous opioids to cholecystokinin. Progress in Neurobiology 52(2):109–125.

British National Formulary (BNF) (2005) London: British Medical Association and Royal Pharmaceutical Society of Great Britain. Available online at www.bnf.org (accessed May 2005).

Committee on Safety of Medicines. Available online at http://medicines.mhra.gov.uk/aboutagency/regframework/csm/csmhome.htm (accessed May 2005).

Electronic Medicines Compendium. Available online at http://www.emc.medicines.org.uk (accessed May 2005).

Hróbjartsson A, Götzsche PC (2001) Is the placebo powerless? An analysis of clinical trials comparing placebo with no treatment. New England Journal of Medicine 344(21):1594–1602.

National Institute for Clinical Excellence (NICE). London, NICE. Available online at www.nice.org.uk (accessed May 2005).

Royal College of Psychiatrists. Available online at www.rcpsych.ac.uk/ (accessed May 2005).

Wright P, Birkett M, David S, et al (2001) Double blind, placebo controlled comparison of intramuscular olanzapine and intramuscular haloperidol in the treatment of acute agitation in schizophrenia. American Journal of Psychiatry 158:1149–1151.

References and further reading

7

Psychotropic drugs for children

Introduction

Psychotropic drugs are frequently used temporarily or indefinitely in the treatment of several psychiatric disorders in children. However, it must be appreciated that children differ from adults in their ability to absorb (usually faster), metabolise (usually faster) and eliminate drugs and psychotropic drugs are not tested extensively in children during clinical development (see Chapter 6). Great care is therefore required when treating children with psychotropic drugs and the Summary of Product Characteristics (SPC) (see Chapter 5) of the drug or a reference such as the British National Formulary (BNF) should always be consulted before doing so.

The disorders for which psychotropic drugs are widely prescribed during childhood may be divided into those that generally first become evident during childhood – nocturnal enuresis, attention deficit hyperactivity disorder (ADHD), autism, sleep disorders, tic disorders and conduct disorder in children with learning disability – and those that more typically manifest during adulthood but that sometimes present during childhood – anxiety disorders (some such as school refusal are very specific to childhood), depression and psychosis.

Nocturnal enuresis

Nocturnal enuresis should be diagnosed only in the absence of organic pathology including urinary tract infection which, although a rare cause of urinary incontinence in boys, should be routinely excluded in girls.

The first-line treatment of nocturnal enuresis is behavioural because this is generally effective. Drug therapy is only appropriate if behavioural treatment proves ineffective or is not possible. Drugs are rarely appropriate for children under the age of 7 years, apart from occasional use to cover periods away from home, for example school trips. Drugs may be used alone or in combination with behavioural treatment.

The drugs used to treat nocturnal enuresis include tricyclic (TCA) antidepressant (AD) drugs, desmopressin and oxybutynin. The need to continue treatment should be determined every 3 months by means of at least 1 week without treatment before a further 3 months of treatment is prescribed. Recurrence is common if these drugs are discontinued and treatment frequently needs to continue for several years.

Tricyclic antidepressant drugs

TCA AD drugs are favoured for the treatment of nocturnal enuresis. Imipramine (0.5–1.0 mg/kg) before going to bed is usually effective within 1–2 weeks and amitriptyline is also effective. The mechanism of action of TCA AD drugs is presumed to involve direct anticholinergic effects on the bladder. The TCA AD drugs are described in detail in Chapter 9.

Desmopressin

Desmopressin (20–40 micrograms) administered orally or by intranasal spray before going to bed is also effective. Desmopressin, a synthetic polypeptide, is a structural analogue of vasopressin. It has a more prolonged antidiuretic effect than vasopressin but significantly less of a vasopressor effect. Its half life ($T_{1/2}$) is 2.5–4.5 hours while its adverse effects include fluid retention, hyponatraemia (which may cause seizures), headache, nausea, vomiting, nasal congestion and rhinitis.

Oxybutynin

Oxybutynin is an antimuscarinic drug that relaxes detrusor smooth muscle. It may be effective in children with treatment-resistant nocturnal enuresis caused by detrusor instability. Such treatment should only be initiated by a specialist following urodynamic studies.

Attention deficit hyperactivity disorder

Attention deficit hyperactivity disorder (ADHD) is diagnosed in 1–2% of UK children and at least 5% of North American children (Swanson et al, 1998). A significant proportion of these children are treated with stimulant medication. This has led to concern that medication is being used to modify childhood behaviour that is within the normal range. This concern is probably unfounded and the behavioural, academic and social response of children with ADHD to effective medication is among the most rapid, dramatic and rewarding in clinical psychopharmacology.

The stimulant drugs licensed for the treatment of ADHD in the UK are methylphenidate, which is widely prescribed, and dexamfetamine, which is prescribed less frequently. Methylphenidate and dexamfetamine are controlled drugs in the UK and both are subject to the prescription requirements of the Misuse of Drugs Regulations 2001. Atomoxetine, a non-stimulant drug which has recently become available, is not a controlled drug.

It should be noted that when children or adults with ADHD are treated with stimulants they become more attentive and less hyperactive and do not develop tolerance. In contrast, individuals who do not have ADHD become less attentive and more hyperactive if they take stimulants, and they quickly develop tolerance.

Approximately 60% of children with ADHD continue to suffer with it in adulthood. The psychotropic drug treatment of ADHD in adults is similar to that employed in children.

Methylphenidate

Pharmacokinetics and pharmacodynamics

Methylphenidate is rapidly absorbed from the gastrointestinal tract and protein binding is low. First pass hepatic metabolism is extensive and elimination is rapid, providing a T_{MAX} of 2 hours and a $T_{1/2}$ of approximately 3 hours. Clinical effects are evident within 1 hour and are of approximately 5 hours' duration. The drug must be administered 3–4 times daily because of its pharmacokinetic parameters. An extended release formulation is available.

Methylphenidate, like dexamfetamine, causes the release of dopamine (DA) and, to a lesser extent, noradrenaline (NA; norepinephrine), from mesocortical (especially prefrontal) and striatal presynaptic neurons (Fig. 7.1). It also blocks the reuptake of DA via the presynaptic DA reuptake transporter protein to these neurones. This presumed mechanism of action is similar to that of cocaine.

Efficacy

Methylphenidate is administered in a dosage of 0.3–0.7 mg per kg per day in children to a maximum of 60 mg daily. Adults respond to doses in the range 20–60 mg daily. It is usually commenced at a dose of 5 mg twice daily and increased every 3–4 days until a beneficial effect is obtained or adverse effects prevent further dose increase. It is rarely

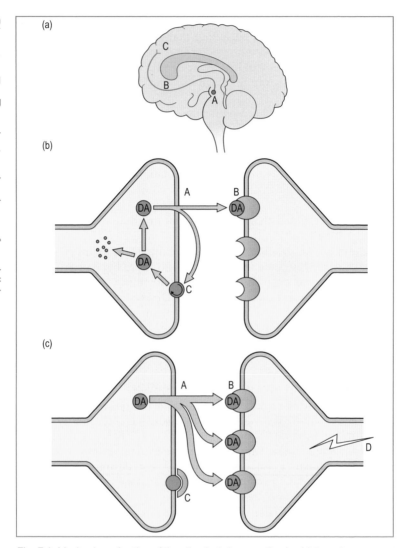

Fig. 7.1 Mechanism of action of the stimulant drugs methyphenidate and dexamfetamine. (**a**) Methylphenidate and dexamfetamine primarily promote the activity of dopaminergic neurones that originate in the ventral tegmental nucleus of the midbrain (A) and project via mesocortical fibres (B) to prefrontal (C) areas.
(**b**) Dopamine (DA) is released from the presynaptic neurone (A) and either binds to postsynaptic DA receptors (B) or re-enters the presynaptic neurone via the reuptake transporter protein (C). (**c**) Methylphenidate and dexamfetamine promote DA release from the presynaptic neurone (A) and block its reuptake via the transporter protein (C). These two actions increase synaptic DA concentration, promote DA binding to postsynaptic receptors (B) and facilitate neuronal firing (D).

necessary to dose above 60 mg per day. A long-acting formulation of methylphenidate that is administered once daily in a dose range of 18–54 mg has recently become available.

Most children with ADHD respond rapidly and significantly to methylphenidate or similar drugs. For example, Elia et al (1991) reported that 96% of children showed behavioural improvement, while a recent review of clinical trials by Greenhill et al (1999) concluded that stimulants such as methylphenidate 'show robust short-term efficacy and a good safety profile'. Indeed response to methylphenidate is so rapid and so reliable in ADHD that a 'trial of treatment' may be undertaken when diagnosis is in doubt.

Methylphenidate also remains effective in the long term. However, the effect of treating ADHD during childhood and adolescence with methylphenidate and other stimulants on eventual adult function is unclear. Methylphenidate is recommended by the National Institute for Health and Clinical Excellence (NICE, 2000):

'...for use as part of a comprehensive treatment programme for children with a diagnosis of severe attention deficit hyperactivity disorder...'

However, clinical trials do not, in fact, provide convincing evidence that educational or behavioural treatment programmes provide additional benefits over and above medications alone (MTA Cooperative Group, 1999). Indeed Taylor (1999) has stated that behavioural treatment alone is unlikely to be effective and that medication should always be considered.

Children whose ADHD has responded to methylphenidate will require prolonged treatment and may benefit from so-called drug-holidays during which treatment is suspended, partly as a means of assessing the need for continuing medication.

Safety

The adverse effects commonly associated with methylphenidate include nervousness, insomnia, urticaria, fever, rash (which may progress to exfoliative dermatitis and erythema multiforme), anorexia, nausea, dizziness, palpitations, headache, dyskinesia, drowsiness, hypertension, tachycardia, angina, abdominal pain and weight loss.

Organic psychosis may occur and abuse and diversion for recreational use are recognised. Greenhill et al (1999) reported no evidence of harmful effects from prolonged treatment on the basis of a literature review.

Methylphenidate should not be prescribed in combination with monoamine oxidase inhibitors (MAOIs) or within 2 weeks after discontinuing treatment with such drugs.

Dexamfetamine

Pharmacokinetics and pharmacodynamics

The presumed mechanism of action of dexamfetamine is similar to that of methylphenidate (see above).

Efficacy

The efficacy of dexamfetamine is similar to that of methylphenidate. However, it should be regarded as an alternative treatment for children who do not respond to methylphenidate, rather than as a first-line treatment. This is because it carries a significant risk of dependence and organic psychosis. Dexamfetamine is only available in the UK in 5 mg tablets and prescriptions may involve several hundreds of tablets. It is administered in a dosage of 5–20 mg per day with a maximum dosage of 40 mg per day in older children and adolescents.

Safety

The adverse effects commonly associated with dexamfetamine include insomnia, irritability, euphoria, tremor, headache, seizures, organic psychosis, anorexia, growth retardation (height should be monitored), hypertension, dry mouth, tachycardia and sweating. Tics and Gilles de la Tourette syndrome have been reported. Organic psychosis may occur and dependence, tolerance and diversion for recreational use are recognised.

Dexamfetamine should not be prescribed in combination with MAOIs or within 2 weeks after discontinuing treatment with such drugs.

Atomoxetine

Pharmacokinetics and pharmacodynamics

Atomoxetine is rapidly absorbed from the gastrointestinal tract and is 98% protein bound. Hepatic metabolism is via the cytochrome P450 CYP 2D6 pathway. The T_{MAX} is 2 hours while the $T_{1/2}$ is approximately 4 hours in extensive metabolisers but is increased to 20 hours in the 5–10% of the population that are poor metabolisers.

Atomoxetine is a highly selective inhibitor of the presynaptic NA reuptake transporter protein but has minimal affinity for other NA receptors (Fig. 7.2). It increases synaptic concentrations of NA in the prefrontal cortex but has no effect on serotonin levels.

Efficacy

Atomoxetine may be administered to children and adolescents under 70 kg in bodyweight in an initial dose of 0.5 mg per kg per day. This may be increased after 3 days to 1.2 mg per kg per day. The total daily dose may be administered as a single dose or as two equal doses. Most

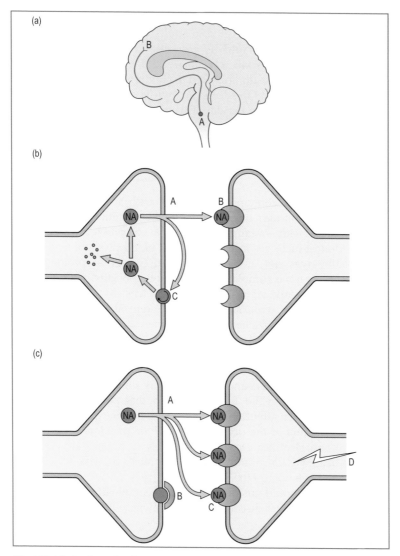

Fig. 7.2 Mechanism of action of the non-stimulant drug atomoxetine.
(**a**) Atomoxetine promotes the activity of noradrenergic neurones that originate in the locus ceruleus (A) and project to the prefrontal cortex (B). (**b**) Noradrenaline (NA; norepinephrine) is released from the presynaptic neurone (A) and either binds to postsynaptic NA receptors (B) or re-enters the presynaptic neurone via the reuptake transporter protein (C). (**c**) Atomoxetine has no effect on NA release from the prepsynaptic neurone (A) but it blocks its reuptake via the transporter protein (B). This action increases synaptic NA concentration, promotes NA binding to postsynaptic receptors (C) and facilitates neuronal firing (D).

children with ADHD respond significantly to atomoxetine and its efficacy has also been established in adults with ADHD. Response to atomoxetine is not as rapid as response to methylphenidate or dexamfetamine and may take several weeks.

Atomoxetine may be administered to children and adolescents over 70 kg in bodyweight, and to adults (unapproved indication in the UK), in an initial dose of 40 mg per day. This may be increased after 3 days to 80 mg per day and, if necessary, after 2 weeks to 100 mg per day.

Individuals whose ADHD has responded to atomoxetine will require prolonged treatment.

Safety

The adverse effects commonly associated with atomoxetine include dry mouth, insomnia, nausea, decreased appetite, constipation, dizziness, headache, sweating, dysuria, sexual problems and palpitations. Modest increases in heart rate and blood pressure may occur. Atomoxetine was not associated with QT interval prolongation. Atomoxetine is not a stimulant and was not associated with abuse or diversion for recreational use during clinical trials.

The dose of atomoxetine should be reduced to 50% of the usual dose in patients with moderate hepatic insufficiency and to 25% of the usual in patients with severe hepatic insufficiency. The Committee on Safety of Medicines (CSM) wrote to doctors and pharmacists in February 2005 advising that 1 in 50,000 patients treated with atomoxetine may develop hepatic disorders and that these may sometimes be severe. In September 2005, the CSM further advised that patients and carers should seek medical attention if abdominal pain, unexplained nausea, malaise, darkening of the urine or jaundice occur. More recently, the Medicines and Healthcare products Regulatory Agency advised that children treated with atomoxetine are at increased risk of suicidal thoughts and behaviour (2005).

Atomoxetine should not be prescribed in combination with MAOIs or within 2 weeks after discontinuing treatment with such drugs.

Other treatments

The TCA AD drugs imipramine and desipramine are occasionally used to treat children with ADHD. Adverse effects are problematic but they may represent a useful alternative to methylphenidate for some patients. Clonidine, an α_2 NA receptor agonist, is also occasionally used as a second-line treatment or as an adjunct to stimulants.

Other AD and occasionally antipsychotic (AP) drugs may also be effective for some patients. Bupropion, carbamazepine and combination treatment with two or more drugs are occasionally employed. The use of such treatments should only be initiated by a specialist.

Psychopharmacology and our understanding of ADHD

The first-line drugs used to treat ADHD primarily increase synaptic concentrations of DA in the case of methylphenidate and dexamfetamine and NA in the case of atomoxetine. This suggests that insufficient DA and NA activity may be responsible for inattention and/or hyperactivity. Human functional neuroimaging and primate lesion studies confirm this suggestion and point to the importance of mesocortical, especially prefrontal, DA and NA neuronal circuits in attention and motivation.

Autism

Psychotropic drugs play a modest but useful role in the alleviation of symptoms associated with autism. Thus:

- atypical AP drugs, usually in low dosage, may help in the short-term treatment of agitation or aggression
- stimulants and atomoxetine may help when ADHD symptoms are present, although they may worsen stereotypies and tic disorders
- antiepileptic drugs (AEDs) are essential when autism coexists with epilepsy and
- selective serotonin reuptake inhibitor (SSRI) AD drugs may help in the management of anxiety, agitation and stereotypic behaviours (but see below for CSM advice).

Few clinical trials have been undertaken in autism and it is impossible to offer definitive advice.

Sleep disorders

Reassurance, education and behavioural treatment rather than psychotropic drugs are the mainstay of the management of sleep disorders in children. Sedating antihistamines such as alimemazine (trimeprazine) 2 mg per kg daily, chloral hydrate 30–50 mg per kg daily and diazepam 0.1–0.3 mg per kg daily are occasionally prescribed for brief periods. Diazepam 0.1–0.3 mg per kg daily or paroxetine 20–40 mg daily are very occasionally prescribed for night terrors.

Tic disorders

The motor and vocal tics of Gilles de la Tourette syndrome typically present during childhood. The syndrome is commoner in children with autism, obsessive compulsive disorder and ADHD than in otherwise healthy children.

Haloperidol, pimozide, clonidine and sulpiride are established treatments and atypical AP drugs and SSRI AD drugs are also used (but see below for CSM advice). Doses of haloperidol should commence at 0.5–1.0 mg three times daily and be slowly increased until a response is obtained. Daily doses as high as 10 mg per day may be required. Clonidine should be titrated to a maximum dose of 10 micrograms per kg per day.

Conduct disorders

The use of psychotropic drugs for the primary purpose of controlling behaviour in children with learning disability is generally inappropriate. These drugs are associated with adverse effects which cause distress, impair cognition and may worsen the behaviour for which they were originally prescribed. Environmental management and psychological therapies are therefore the preferred treatments for such individuals. Psychotropic drugs should only be prescribed for children with learning disability when the primary purpose is either the short-term control of a crisis or the long-term treatment of a psychiatric disorder such as schizophrenia or depression.

AP drugs are widely prescribed for the control of agitation, self-harming and aggression in children with learning disability. Such individuals have brain damage by definition and are therefore at great risk of developing extrapyramidal adverse effects if treated with typical AP drugs. Extrapyramidal adverse effects, especially akathisia, may exacerbate rather than reduce agitation and aggression. Atypical AP drugs should therefore be the first choice if it is necessary to prescribe AP drugs for children with learning disability. They are being increasingly used for this purpose and should be prescribed in the lowest effective dose for the shortest duration of time necessary. Children with learning disability who have a psychotic disorder (at least 2% of such individuals have schizophrenia, for example) may benefit from prolonged treatment with atypical AP drugs.

AEDs are also widely prescribed for children with learning disability, both in the treatment of epilepsy and recurrent mood disorders and in an attempt to reduce episodes of disturbed behaviour. Their use in the latter situation should only be commenced with recording of the target behaviour before and during treatment and with great attention to adverse effects. AEDs should be discontinued if the benefit/risk balance proves unfavourable.

SSRI AD drugs may help children with learning disability who have depression and may also reduce the frequency and severity of self-harming in some such individuals (but see below for CSM advice). Stimulant medications and atomoxetine may be beneficial if ADHD is present.

Anxiety

SSRI AD drugs, especially fluoxetine and sertraline, may be useful in the treatment of anxiety disorders, including obsessive compulsive disorder, in childhood (but see below for CSM advice).

Psychotropic medication has no place in the management of school refusal unless there is an underlying psychiatric disorder such as anxiety or depression present.

Depression

SSRI AD drugs have become the mainstay of the treatment of children with depression. Older AD drugs are largely avoided because of their adverse effects.

The CSM issued a Dear Doctor Letter (see Chapter 5) about the use of SSRI AD drugs in children in December 2004. This states that the balance of benefits and risks of such drugs in the treatment of individuals under the age of 18 years is only favourable for fluoxetine.

Psychosis

Psychotic disorders are rare in childhood. When they occur, their treatment is the same as during adulthood. Thus atypical AP drugs should be prescribed at low dosage and the dose slowly titrated upwards until a response is obtained. The successful use of clozapine in children with treatment-resistant psychosis has been reported.

References and further reading

Committee on Safety of Medicines. Strattera (atomoxetine) – risk of hepatic disorders. CEM/CMO/2005. Available online at http://medicines.mhra.gov.uk/aboutagency/regframework/csm/csmhome.htm (accessed May 2005).

Committee on Safety of Medicines. Safety of selective serotonin reuptake inhibitor antidepressants CEM/CMO/2004/11. Available online at http://medicines.mhra.gov.uk/aboutagency/regframework/csm/csmhome.htm (accessed June 2005).

Committee on Safety of Medicines www.mca.gov.uk/aboutagency/regframework/csm/csmhome.htm (accessed October 2005).

Elia J, Borcherding BG, Rapoport JL, Keysor CS (1991) Methylphenidate and dextroamphetamine treatments of hyperactivity: are there true nonresponders? Psychiatry Research 36(2):141–155.

Greenhill LL, Halperin JM, Abikoff H (1999) Stimulant medications. Journal of the American Academy of Child and Adolescent Psychiatry 38(5): 503–512.

Medicines and Healthcare products Regulatory Agency http://www.mhra.gov.uk/ (accessed October 2005).

MTA Cooperative Group (1999) A 14-month randomized clinical trial of treatment strategies for attention-deficit/hyperactivity disorder. Multimodal Treatment Study of Children with ADHD. Archives of General Psychiatry 56(12):1073–1086.

National Institute for Clinical Excellence (2000) Guidance on the Use of Methylphenidate for ADHD (www.nice.org.uk) (accessed October 2005).

Swanson JM, Sergeant JA, Taylor E, Sonuga-Barke EJ, Jensen PS, Cantwell DP (1998) Attention-deficit hyperactivity disorder and hyperkinetic disorder. Lancet 351:429–433.

Taylor E (1999) Development of clinical services for attention-deficit/hyperactivity disorder. Archives of General Psychiatry 56(12):1097–1099.

8

Antipsychotic drugs

Introduction

Antipsychotic (AP) drugs are conventionally divided into two classes, the newer atypical and the older typical AP drugs. The principal difference between these two classes is that patients are much less likely to experience extrapyramidal system (EPS) adverse effects with atypical than with typical AP drugs. The atypical AP drugs include:

- three dibenzazepines – clozapine (a dibenzodiazepine), olanzapine (a thienobenzodiazepine) and quetiapine (a dibenzothiazepine) and
- several drugs with diverse structures – amisulpride (a substituted benzamide), aripiprazole (a quinolinone derivative), risperidone (a benzisoxazole), sertindole (an indole derivative), ziprasidone (a benzothiazoylpiperazine) and zotepine (a dibenzothiepine).

Clozapine may be regarded as the archetypal atypical AP drug.

The typical AP drugs include the butyrophenones such as haloperidol, the phenothiazines such as chlorpromazine and the thioxanthines such as flupenthixol.

Haloperidol may be regarded as the archetypal typical AP drug.

All of the AP drugs listed above are first-line treatments for schizophrenia and similar psychoses with the exception of clozapine and sertindole, which are second-line treatments (see below). Ziprasidone is not available in the UK.

Pharmacokinetics

The pharmacokinetics (PK) of orally administered and injectable AP drugs differ from each other and must be considered separately.

Orally administered antipsychotic drugs

The AP drugs have relatively similar pharmacokinetics (PK). In general therefore, AP drugs that are administered as tablets:

* are rapidly and completely absorbed at the proximal small intestine with T_{MAX} ranging from 1–5 hours
* are subject to extensive first pass metabolism
* have plasma protein binding in excess of 90%
* are metabolised almost exclusively in the liver
* are metabolised almost completely (almost no parent drug is excreted) and
* have $T_{1/2}$ that range from 0.5–3 days in duration (the $T_{1/2}$ of depot formulations may extend over some months – see below).

Some AP drugs are available in liquid (risperidone, for example) or orodispersible (olanzapine and risperidone, for example) formulations. The PK of these formulations are similar to those of tablets.

Injectable antipsychotic drugs

A few atypical and several typical AP drugs are available as rapidly acting intramuscular (IM) injections for the treatment of agitation and disturbed behaviours or as depot injections for the long-term treatment of psychotic illness.

Rapidly acting intramuscular formulations

Olanzapine is the only atypical AP available in a rapidly acting IM formulation in the UK. Its pharmacokinetics differ from those of olanzapine tablets in that T_{MAX} is reached after 30–40 minutes rather than after 3–4 hours and C_{MAX} is 3–4 times greater than for the same dose administered orally. The $T_{1/2}$ of both IM and oral olanzapine is similar. Rapidly acting IM ziprasidone is available in some countries and a similar formulation of aripiprazole is being developed.

Depot injections

The PK of depot formulations of AP drugs differ from those of tablets in that release from the injection site in muscle to the systemic circulation is delayed by use of an oily solvent and/or esterification of the drug. A clinically insignificant proportion of drug enters the systemic circulation immediately after injection but therapeutic blood levels are not achieved for some days. Once achieved, such levels persist for 6 weeks or longer.

Risperidone is the only atypical AP drug currently available in depot formulation in the UK. A clinically insignificant proportion of depot risperidone enters the systemic circulation immediately after injection but clinically effective blood levels are not achieved for approximately 3 weeks after injection. Supplementation with oral risperidone is therefore necessary for approximately 3 weeks following the initial injection. Therapeutic blood levels are maintained for approximately 4–6 weeks after subsequent injections and drug is cleared from the body after approximately 8 weeks. Depot formulations of olanzapine and aripiprazole are being developed.

Pharmacodynamics

It is convenient to separate the mesolimbic dopaminergic system from the three other dopaminergic systems when considering the pharmacodynamics of AP drugs (see Chapter 3).

Mesolimbic dopaminergic systems

The affinity of AP drugs, both atypical and typical, for postsynaptic DA D_2 receptors in the mesolimbic system appears to determine their efficacy (Fig. 8.1). Thus blockade of these postsynaptic DA D_2 receptors by AP drugs prevents DA from exerting its agonist effect and reduces the excess dopaminergic activity in the mesolimbic system that is implicated in schizophrenia. The affinity of AP drugs for postsynaptic DA D_2 receptors may be measured *in vitro* in brain tissue, and *in vivo* in animals, using radiolabelled ligands. Raclopride labelled with ^3H, for example, binds with reasonable specificity to DA D_2 receptors. AP drugs occupy these receptors and inhibit binding by ^3H raclopride. Measurements of radioactivity before and after administration of AP drugs therefore allow their affinity for the receptor to be calculated. This process generates data such as those presented in Table 8.1 in which the numbers represent the dose of AP drug in mg/kg that produces an effect in 50% of the samples studied, the ED_{50} (Zhang and Bymaster, 2000). It will be appreciated that the lower the ED_{50}, the greater the affinity of the AP drug for the receptor. Haloperidol, for example, with an ED_{50} of 0.12 mg/kg, has the greatest affinity for DA D_2 receptors.

Functional neuroimaging studies, both positron emission tomography (PET) and single photon emission tomography (SPET), in patients with schizophrenia are in keeping with *in vitro* and *in vivo* studies in that they demonstrate that all effective AP drugs, atypical and typical, have a relatively high, and in many cases dose-dependent, affinity for DA D_2 receptors. Unfortunately however, this finding is most readily demonstrated for striatal presynaptic, rather than mesolimbic or mesocortical postsynaptic, DA D_2 receptors. Binding of ^{11}C raclopride to striatal DA D_2 receptors, for example, is inhibited by ziprasidone (see Fig. 8.2). Thus this finding tells us more about how AP drugs cause EPS adverse effects than about their beneficial mechanism of action. However, more recent work with ^{18}F fallypride indicates that while olanzapine and haloperidol occupy DA D_2 receptors in striatum, thalamus, amygdala and temporal cortex to a similar extent (70% approximately), olanzapine occupancy of DA D_2 receptors in the substantia nigra is significantly lower than that of haloperidol (40% versus 70% approximately) (Kessler et al, 2005). It will be appreciated

Table 8.1: Inhibition of radioligand binding to neuroreceptors by selected atypical AP drugs and haloperidol (ED_{50} values mg/kg)

	D_1	D_2	$5HT_2$	Muscarinic
Clozapine	70	20	2.2	>30
Olanzapine	15	0.6	0.15	10
Quetiapine	>40	25	7	>40
Risperidone	>3	0.2	0.1	>3
Sertindole	>10	4.2	0.2	>10
Ziprasidone	>30	5	0.5	>30
Haloperidol	>10	0.12	1.6	>3

Fig. 8.1 (*Facing page*) Mechanism of action of the typical antipsychotic drugs in the treatment of schizophrenia and other psychotic disorders. (**a**) Typical antipsychotic drugs primarily affect the mesolimbic, mesocortical, nigrostriatal and tuberoinfundibular dopaminergic systems. (**b**) Excessive dopaminergic (DA) activity in the mesolimbic system is thought to underpin the positive symptoms of schizophrenia while insufficient dopaminergic activity in the mesocortical, nigrostriatal and tuberoinfundibular dopaminergic systems is thought respectively to underpin negative symptoms and cognitive dysfunction in schizophrenia, and the extrapyramidal system (EPS) adverse effects and hyperprolactinaemia associated with typical antipsychotic drugs. (**c**) Blockade of postsynaptic DA D_2 receptors in the mesolimbic system reduces excessive dopaminergic activity and alleviates the positive symptoms of schizophrenia. However, blockade of such receptors in the mesocortical, nigrostriatal and tuberoinfundibular systems may exacerbate negative symptoms and cognitive dysfunction, and cause EPS adverse effects and hyperprolactinaemia.

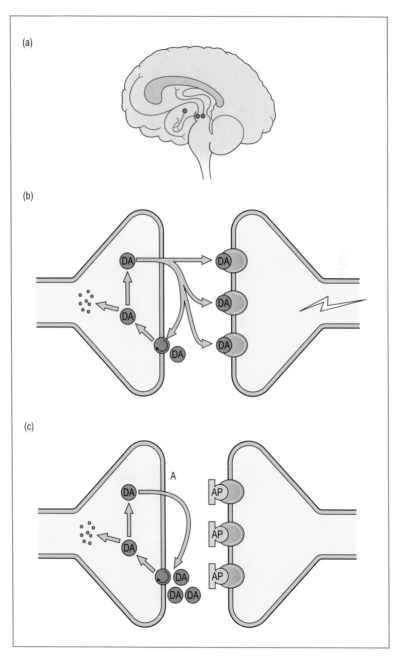

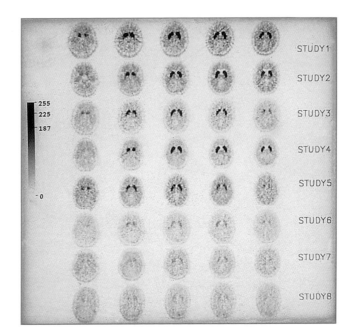

Fig. 8.2 PET images of ^{11}C raclopride, a dopamine D_2 receptor ligand. The images are darkest in the striatum where the highest levels of ^{11}C raclopride occurs. Subject study 4 received placebo, and subject studies 1–3 and 5–8 received increasing doses of ziprasidone (2, 5, 10, 15, 20, 40 and 60 mg). The images show decreasing binding of ^{11}C raclopride due to ziprasidone's increasing occupancy of the dopamine D_2 receptor. (Image courtesy of Dr C Bench, MRC Cyclotron Unit, Hammersmith Hospital, London.)

that this finding may explain why atypical AP drugs carry a lower risk of EPS adverse effects than typical AP drugs.

A fast dissociation hypothesis of AP efficacy and safety has recently been proposed for the atypical AP drug, aripiprazole (Kapur and Seeman, 2001). This proposes that while D_2 receptor occupancy produces the drug's antipsychotic effect, it is its rapid dissociation from the D_2 receptor, rather than lower affinity for it or occupancy of $5HT_{2A}$ or other receptors, that accounts for its EPS safety.

The atypical and typical AP drugs differ significantly in their affinity for mesolimbic postsynaptic D_2 receptors (see Table 8.2). It is effectively impossible to occupy all such receptors with atypical AP drugs, even when administered in very high doses. In contrast, almost all receptors are occupied following modest doses of typical AP drugs. This has led to the view that while occupancy of approximately 70% of mesolimbic postsynaptic D_2 receptors is necessary and sufficient for

Table 8.2: Relative *in vivo* occupancy of postsynaptic D_2 receptors by selected atypical AP drugs and haloperidol measured by inhibition of radioligand binding to receptors

	% D_2 receptor binding
Clozapine	50
Olanzapine	70
Quetiapine	59
Risperidone	81
Sertindole	68
Ziprasidone	85
Haloperidol	99

the antipsychotic efficacy of atypical and typical AP drugs, occupancy above this level may be responsible for adverse effects (see below).

It is generally thought that the antipsychotic efficacy of AP drugs only becomes evident after some weeks. This delayed onset of action is thought to reflect both the time taken to reach steady state and post-receptor events such as long-term potentiation. However, the very existence of delayed onset of antipsychotic efficacy has recently been questioned (Wright et al, 2003).

Other dopaminergic systems

The affinity of AP drugs for postsynaptic D_2 receptors in the frontal cortex, basal ganglia and tuberoinfundibular system appears to determine their adverse effects. It is thought that blockade of the cortical postsynaptic D_2 receptors with which dopaminergic fibres extending from the ventral tegmental nucleus synapse by typical AP drugs may be responsible for some of the negative and cognitive symptoms of schizophrenia. Thus such symptoms may be iatrogenic to some extent (see below).

The affinity of AP drugs for postsynaptic D_2 receptors in the basal ganglia appears to determine their EPS safety. These are the receptors with which dopaminergic fibres extending from the substantia nigra synapse. Atypical AP drugs may have significantly less affinity for these nigrostriatal D_2 receptors than typical AP drugs (see above).

DA inhibits the release of prolactin from the pituitary gland. Blockade of postsynaptic D_2 receptors in the tuberoinfundibular system prevents this inhibitory effect of DA and causes hyper-prolactinaemia (see below).

Atypical AP drugs have relatively high affinities for $5HT_{2A}$ receptors (see Table 8.1). Physiologically, $5HT_{2A}$ receptors occur on the cell bodies and terminal axon fibres of DA neurones in the frontal cortex, basal ganglia and tuberoinfundibular system. Occupancy of these receptors by 5HT inhibits the release of DA into the synapse (Fig. 8.3). Blockade of these receptors by atypical AP drugs prevents 5HT from exerting its inhibitory effect and increases dopaminergic activity in the frontal cortex, basal ganglia and tuberoinfundibular system. This mechanism may account in part for the reduction in negative and cognitive symptoms, in EPS adverse effects and in hyper-prolactinaemia associated with atypical AP drugs.

Psychopharmacology and our understanding of psychosis

The effects of psychotomimetic drugs that are misused, such as amfetamine and cocaine, and of AP drugs that are prescribed, has contributed significantly to our understanding of schizophrenia in particular, and of psychosis in general.

The dopamine hypothesis of schizophrenia

It has long been observed that drugs that increase dopaminergic activity in the brain may cause positive symptoms of schizophrenia such as hallucinations and delusions in non-schizophrenic individuals, and may exacerbate symptoms in patients with schizophrenia. Thus:

Fig. 8.3 (*Facing page*) Mechanism of action of the atypical antipsychotic drugs in the treatment of schizophrenia and other psychotic disorders. (**a**) Atypical antipsychotic (AP) drugs primarily affect the mesolimbic, mesocortical, nigrostriatal and tuberoinfundibular dopaminergic systems. Their mechanism of action in the mesolimbic system is identical to that of typical antipsychotic drugs (see Fig. 8.1). (**b**) Physiologically, $5HT_{2A}$ receptors occur on the cell bodies (not shown) and terminal axon fibres of DA neurones in the frontal cortex, basal ganglia and tuberoinfundibular systems. Occupancy of these receptors by 5HT inhibits the release of DA into the synapse. Insufficient mesocortical dopaminergic activity is thought to underpin negative symptoms and cognitive dysfunction in schizophrenia while blockade of postsynaptic nigrostriatal and tuberoinfundibular DA D_2 receptors by typical antipsychotic drugs may mediate the extrapyramidal system (EPS) adverse effects and hyperprolactinaemia associated with them. (**c**) Blockade of $5HT_{2A}$ receptors on the cell bodies and terminal axon fibres of DA neurones in the frontal cortex, basal ganglia and tuberoinfundibular systems by atypical AP drugs prevents 5HT from exerting its inhibitory effect and increases dopaminergic activity in the frontal cortex, basal ganglia and tuberoinfundibular system. This mechanism may account in part for the reduction in negative and cognitive symptoms, in EPS adverse effects and in hyperprolactinaemia associated with atypical AP drugs.

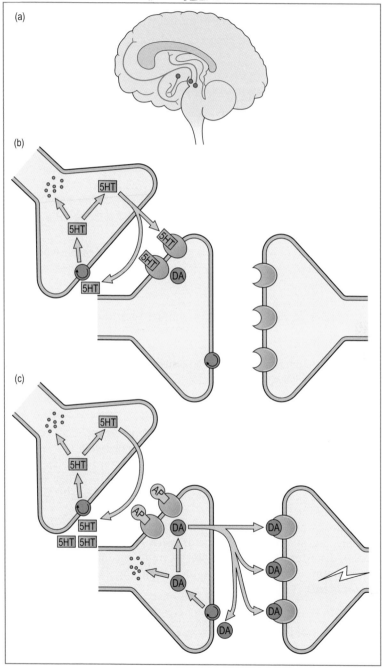

- amfetamine and cocaine which cause DA release at the synapse produce persecutory delusions in non-schizophrenic individuals
- levodopa which increases central DA concentrations causes auditory hallucinations in non-schizophrenic individuals and
- disulfiram which inhibits dopamine metabolism exacerbates the symptoms of patients with schizophrenia.

These observations underpin the DA hypothesis of schizophrenia. This states that schizophrenia is caused by excess dopaminergic activity in mesolimbic and mesocortical brain regions. The DA hypothesis is further supported by the observation that:

- all effective antipsychotic drugs are potent DA D_2 receptor antagonists
- antipsychotic efficacy correlates significantly with DA D_2 receptor occupancy and
- only the α isomer of flupenthixol is a DA D_2 receptor antagonist and an effective antipsychotic; the β isomer is not a D_2 antagonist and is clinically inactive.

A number of research findings conflict with the DA hypothesis. Thus:

- amfetamine, cocaine, levodopa and disulfiram produce only positive, and never negative, schizophrenic symptoms
- AP drugs block DA D_2 receptors within hours of administration but antipsychotic efficacy is not apparent for days or weeks (see above) and
- AP drugs are ineffective in about 30% of patients with schizophrenia, despite their causing 'adequate' DA D_2 receptor blockade.

However, the fact that all effective antipsychotic drugs without exception are potent DA D_2 receptor antagonists is generally regarded as 'proof' of the DA hypothesis.

AP drugs are not 'anti-schizophrenic' and they also effectively alleviate the symptoms of patients with other psychoses such as bipolar disorder. It may therefore be more accurate to talk of the DA hypothesis of psychosis rather than the DA hypothesis of schizophrenia.

The serotonin hypothesis of schizophrenia

The 5HT hypothesis states that schizophrenia is caused by excess serotonergic activity in the brain. It is based on the following key observations:

- lysergic acid diethylamine (LSD) and psilocybin which are $5HT_{2A/2C}$ receptor agonists cause positive symptoms of schizophrenia in non-schizophrenic individuals and
- several atypical AP drugs are potent $5HT_{2A}$ receptor antagonists.

However, LSD generally produces visual hallucinations and these are uncommon in schizophrenia. Furthermore, typical AP drugs are also $5HT_{2A}$ receptor antagonists, albeit not as potent as atypical AP drugs. And of course all atypical AP drugs are potent D_2 receptor antagonists.

Recent investigations suggest that midbrain serotonergic neurones may modulate dopaminergic systems in the limbic system, the cortex and the basal ganglia. Several newer antipsychotics have greater affinity at the $5HT_{2A/2C}$ receptor than at the D_2 receptor.

The excitatory amino acid hypothesis of schizophrenia

The major excitatory amino acids (EAAs) are glutamate and aspartate. The EAA hypothesis states that schizophrenia is caused by insufficient EAAs or their kainate, quisqualate or N-methyl-D-aspartate (NMDA) receptors (see Chapter 3). The hypothesis is supported by reports of:

- low cerebrospinal fluid levels of glutamate in patients with schizophrenia
- reduced numbers of kainate, quisqualate and NMDA receptors in the temporal cortex of patients with schizophrenia and
- the development of positive and negative symptoms of schizophrenia in non-schizophrenic individuals, and exacerbations of illness in patients with schizophrenia, following the administration of a single dose of phencyclidine (PCP), a non-competitive NMDA receptor antagonist.

Efficacy

The psychiatric disorders that the AP drugs currently available in the UK are indicated to treat are presented in Table 8.3 (indications differ depending on when the drug was approved and which regulatory process was followed – see Chapter 5).

AP drugs are generally effective:

- in treating acute exacerbations of schizophrenia, manic episode and other acute psychoses
- in preventing relapse in patients with schizophrenia and other psychoses and
- in preventing relapse in patients with bipolar disease when mood stabilising drugs are ineffective or are not tolerated.

Table 8.3: The approved indications of the atypical AP drugs currently available in the UK and of haloperidol, a representative typical AP drug

Neurotransmitter class	Neurotransmitter	
Dibenzazepines	Clozapine	Schizophrenia – treatment resistant or when severe EPS adverse effects occur; Psychosis in Parkinson's disease
	Olanzapine	Schizophrenia – acute (including agitation/disturbed behaviour), maintenance; Bipolar disorder – manic episode (including agitation/disturbed behaviour), maintenance
	Quetiapine	Schizophrenia; Manic episode
Drugs with diverse structures	Amisulpride	Schizophrenia – acute, maintenance
	Aripiprazole	Schizophrenia
	Risperidone	Schizophrenia – acute, maintenance; Other psychoses; Manic episode
	Sertindole	Schizophrenia – when adverse effects occur with ≥ 1 other AP drug
	Zotepine	Schizophrenia
Typical AP drugs	Haloperidol	Schizophrenia – acute, maintenance (including children); Other psychoses; Manic episode; Aggression and hyperactivity (including children), self-mutilation; Agitation, excitement, violent or dangerously impulsive behaviour; Restlessness and agitation in the elderly; Gilles de la Tourette syndrome (including children) and severe tics

Schizophrenia

It is generally accepted that all AP drugs are equally effective in alleviating the positive symptoms of schizophrenia and in treating other acute psychoses such as manic episode and organic psychosis. There is some evidence that atypical AP drugs, particularly clozapine, are more effective than typical AP drugs in alleviating the negative symptoms of schizophrenia and in reducing depressive symptoms, suicidal behaviour and completed suicide (Meltzer et al, 2003; Wright and O'Flaherty, 2003). More recent evidence suggests that atypical AP drugs such as olanzapine and risperidone may also improve cognitive function in patients with schizophrenia (Bilder et al, 2002). Whether they accomplish this directly, by cognitive enhancement, or indirectly, by causing less cognitive impairment than typical AP drugs, is at present unclear. More recently, a magnetic resonance imaging study of patients with first episode psychosis reported a further difference between the atypical and typical AP drugs (Lieberman et al, 2005). Thus while haloperidol caused significant reductions in brain volume, particularly grey matter volume, after 12 months of treatment, olanzapine did not. This may be because of haloperidol-associated neurotoxicity or olanzapine-associated neuroprotection.

Atypical AP drugs have been recommended as the first-line treatment for almost all patients with schizophrenia by the National Institute for Health and Clinical Excellence (NICE) in the UK (2002) (Box 8.1) and other similar authorities. It seems reasonable to extrapolate this recommendation to all other patients who require AP drugs, for example those with acute mania or organic psychosis.

AP drug treatment should commence with an adequate dose of a single atypical AP drug. If this is ineffective after 2–3 weeks the dose should be increased and treatment continued for a further 2–3 weeks. If treatment remains ineffective this drug should be discontinued, a

---

nice guidelines

Box 8.1: National Institute for Health and Clinical Excellence guidance on the use of atypical antipsychotic drugs for the treatment of schizophrenia

1. The atypical AP drugs amisulpride, olanzapine, quetiapine, risperidone and zotepine should be considered when choosing first-line treatment for patients with newly diagnosed schizophrenia.*
2. The atypical AP drugs should be considered the treatment of choice for managing an acute schizophrenic episode when discussion with the patient is not possible.
3. The atypical AP drugs should be considered for a patient who is suffering unacceptable adverse effects from a conventional AP drug.
4. An atypical antipsychotic should be considered for a patient in relapse whose symptoms were previously inadequately controlled.
5. Changing to an atypical AP drug is not necessary if a conventional AP drug controls symptoms adequately and does not cause unacceptable side-effects.
6. Clozapine should be introduced if schizophrenia is inadequately controlled despite the sequential use of two or more AP drugs, one of which should be an atypical AP drug, each for at least 6–8 weeks.

*Aripiprazole had not been approved when this Guidance was published in 2002.

second atypical AP drug should be prescribed and the same two-stage process should be repeated. If the second atypical AP drug proves ineffective treatment with clozapine should be commenced. If the first atypical AP drug is not tolerated the patient should be switched to treatment with the second atypical AP drug. If this is not tolerated the patient should be switched to treatment with clozapine.

Clozapine is used as a second-line AP drug in patients with treatment-resistant schizophrenia. Treatment-resistant schizophrenia may be defined as an inadequate response to two different atypical AP drugs prescribed in adequate doses for an adequate duration of time and/or EPS side effects caused by AP drugs. Patients treated with clozapine require haematological monitoring because of the risk of agranulocytosis (see Table 8.4 and below).

The starting dose, dose range and available formulations of the atypical AP drugs that are currently approved in the UK, and of haloperidol, are presented in Table 8.4.

The relapse rate in untreated schizophrenic patients reaches almost 100% after 2 years. Long-term AP drug therapy is therefore essential for the majority of patients once the acute episode has resolved. Such prophylactic AP treatment should be continued indefinitely in almost all patients because it is clear that the risk of relapse never diminishes. Any patient who insists on discontinuing prophylactic AP treatment should be reviewed regularly and such treatment should be reinstated immediately upon recurrence of psychotic symptoms.

Patients who refuse oral AP therapy or who are agitated may require a parenterally administered AP drug. Parenteral formulations of atypical AP drugs have recently become available and IM olanzapine is reported to reduce agitation as effectively as, but more rapidly than, either IM haloperidol or IM lorazepam (Wright et al, 2003). IM ziprasidone is available in the US and some other countries but not in the UK while IM aripiprazole is being developed. NICE have made the following important recommendations about the treatment of schizophrenic patients who are agitated (2002):

- Oral administration of medication is preferred to parenteral administration on grounds of patient dignity.
- Intramuscular administration of medication is preferred to intravenous administration on grounds of patient safety.
- The intramuscular drugs recommended for use are haloperidol, lorazepam and olanzapine.
- A single drug is preferred to a combination of drugs whenever possible.
- If haloperidol (or another typical antipsychotic drug) is administered intramuscularly, an antimuscarinic drug should also be administered in order to reduce the risk of acute dystonia and other EPS side-effects.

		Oral starting dose (mg)	Oral dose range (mg)	Available formulations
Dibenzazepines	Clozapine*	12.5–25	200–900	Tablets
	Olanzapine	10	5–20	Tablets Orodispersible tablets IM injection
	Quetiapine	50	300–750	Tablets
Drugs with diverse structures	Amisulpride	400–800	400–1200	Tablets Liquid
	Aripiprazole	10	10–30	Tablets
	Risperidone	2	4–16	Tablets Orodispersible tablets Liquid Depot injection
	Sertindole**	4	12–24	Tablets
	Zotepine	75	75–300	Tablets
Typical AP drugs	Haloperidol	3	3–30	Tablets Liquid IM injection Depot injection

*Only prescribers/patients who are registered with CPMS, the Clozaril Patient Monitoring Service, may prescribe/be treated with clozapine.
**Sertindole has been reintroduced following an earlier suspension because of concerns about arrhythmias; its use in the UK is restricted to patients who are enrolled in clinical trials and are intolerant of at least one other AP drug.

The majority of patients with schizophrenia have little or no appreciation of the fact that they are ill. Indeed lack of insight, present in 97% of patients, was the commonest symptom recorded by the International Pilot Study of Schizophrenia (World Health Organization, 1973). Such patients are therefore understandably reluctant to take AP drugs. This, and the adverse effects associated with these drugs, mean that adherence to prophylactic AP drug treatment is problematic. Injectable depot formulations of AP drugs reduce this problem to some extent in that patients may be more wiling to accept an IM injection every few weeks than tablets every day. Until recently, only typical AP drugs were available in depot formulation. More recently, a depot formulation of risperidone has become available in the UK and depot formulations of olanzapine and aripiprazole are being developed. The pharmacokinetics of depot AP drugs differ significantly from those of orally administered AP drugs (see above).

Bipolar disorder

Atypical and typical AP drugs have long been prescribed for patients with acute mania. Such pragmatic treatment has recently been endorsed by the approval of olanzapine, quetiapine and risperidone for the treatment of acute mania.

The relapse rate in patients with untreated bipolar disorder is, if anything, higher than that in patients with untreated schizophrenia. Such patients are frequently treated with AP drugs when mood stabilising drugs are ineffective or are not tolerated. Heretofore, such treatment was prescribed pragmatically. More recently, olanzapine has been approved for the prevention of manic and depressive relapse in patients with bipolar disorder (Tohen et al, 2005). As with schizophrenia, maintenance therapy should be continued indefinitely in such patients because the risk of relapse persists indefinitely.

Other psychoses

It has already been noted that AP drugs are effective not only in schizophrenia and bipolar disorder but also in organic psychosis. They are also generally effective in patients with psychotic symptoms caused by a range of psychiatric and general medical disorders including:

* depression with psychotic symptoms, paranoia, paraphrenia, acute and transient psychoses, induced delusional disorder and
* acute organic psychoses caused by alcohol withdrawal, head injury or dementia, psychoses associated with epilepsy and drug-induced psychoses including those caused by dopamimetic treatments for Parkinson's disease.

Patients with depression with psychotic symptoms respond poorly to monotherapy with antidepressant drugs when compared to patients with depression without psychotic symptoms (Chan et al, 1987). Combination therapy with both antidepressant and AP drugs is an effective treatment for such patients.

The uncommon eponymous (for example de Clerambault's, Othello, Capgras, Ekbom's and Fregoli syndromes) and non-eponymous (for example delusional dysmorphophobia and paranoia querulans) persistent delusional disorders are difficult to treat and patients both comply poorly with, and respond poorly to, AP drugs. Nonetheless, such drugs are widely prescribed for such patients.

Equivalent doses of antipsychotic drugs

It may sometimes be helpful to know the approximate equivalent daily doses of different AP drugs, for example when switching a patient from one to another or when evaluating a patient who is being treated with an AP drug with which one is unfamiliar. Table 8.5 presents the daily doses that provide approximately equivalent AP efficacy for a number of AP drugs. However, it must be appreciated that individuals respond differently to AP drugs, that equivalent doses do not take account of adverse effects and that for some AP drugs, for example quetiapine, titration upwards from a low initial dose may be required. Table 8.5 should therefore only be used as a guideline.

Safety

As noted above, all effective AP drugs have a high affinity for, and are potent antagonists at, DA D_2 receptors. AP drugs also exert an effect at many other neuroreceptors and their adverse effects are caused by their activity at both DA D_2 and these other neuroreceptors (Table 8.6).

Table 8.5: Approximate equivalent daily doses of some antipsychotic drugs

Antipsychotic drug	Daily dose (mg)
Chlorpromazine*	100
Clozapine	50
Olanzapine	5
Quetiapine	250
Risperidone	1
Haloperidol	2

*Chlorpromazine 100 mg daily is generally employed in AP equivalent daily dose calculations for historical reasons.

Table 8.6: Adverse effects attributable to the antagonist effects of AP drugs at different neuroreceptors

Neuroreceptor (effect)	Adverse effect
Dopaminergic D$_2$ (antagonist)	Acute dystonia, akathisia, Parkinsonism, tardive dyskinesia, neuroleptic malignant syndrome, hyperprolactinaemia and its effects
Cholinergic (antagonist)	Dry mouth, constipation (including paralytic ileus in older patients), dry eyes, blurred vision, closed angle glaucoma, urinary hesitancy, urinary retention (especially in males with prostatic hypertrophy), sexual dysfunction, mild tachycardia (caused by reduced vagal tone), impaired memory, confusion
Noradrenergic (antagonist)	Dizziness, postural hypotension (which may be associated with syncope or reflex tachycardia), arrhythmias, sexual dysfunction
Serotonergic (antagonist)	Weight gain
Histaminergic (antagonist)	Weight gain

Atypical AP drugs cause anticholinergic, antiadrenergic, antiserotonergic and antihistaminergic adverse effects but are much less likely to cause antidopaminergic adverse effects than typical AP drugs. All of the adverse effects listed in Table 8.6 occur to a significant extent with all typical AP drugs.

General adverse effects

The general adverse effects of AP drugs are non-specific and may also be caused by other psychotropic drugs. Those listed in Table 8.6 may be attributed to specific neurotransmitter systems with some confidence but the pathophysiology of the remainder is not well understood. In addition to those listed in Table 8.6, the most significant of these general adverse effects are:

- drowsiness (which may be exacerbated by alcohol and other drugs and may affect driving and occupational performance)
- agitation
- headache
- seizures

- metabolic disturbances including hyperglycaemia, diabetes mellitus and dyslipidaemias (see below)
- blood dyscrasias (see below)
- impaired temperature regulation (see below)
- jaundice including cholestatic jaundice
- changes to eyes including corneal and lens opacities and pigmentation of conjunctiva, cornea and retina.

Their safety profile means that AP drugs should be prescribed cautiously in patients with cardiovascular disease, prostatism, epilepsy, Parkinson's disease, hepatic or renal impairment, blood dyscrasias and closed angle glaucoma. AP drugs are relatively contraindicated in patients with impaired consciousness and phaeochromocytoma. Some AP drugs cause photosensitivity and skin sensitisation.

Metabolic adverse events

The metabolic adverse effects associated with AP drugs include weight gain, hyperglycaemia and diabetes mellitus, and dyslipidaemias. All AP drugs, but particularly the dibenzazepines clozapine and olanzapine, are commonly associated with weight gain. This is not dose dependent and may be very significant in some patients. AP-associated weight gain may be prevented or reversed in a significant proportion of patients by educational programmes that encourage appropriate diet and exercise but others will need to switch to an alternative AP drug.

Hyperglycaemia, exacerbation of or development of diabetes mellitus, ketoacidosis, hyperosmolar coma and deaths have been reported following treatment with AP drugs. Schizophrenia and bipolar disorder themselves approximately double the risk of developing diabetes mellitus while treatment with AP drugs approximately doubles it again. Dear Doctor Letters (see Chapter 5) advising of the risk of diabetes mellitus with all atypical AP drugs available in the US were issued in 2004 on the instruction of the Food and Drug Administration. Patients with diabetes mellitus and those with risk factors for it should be monitored carefully for worsening of, or development of, diabetes if they require treatment with AP drugs.

Modest hypercholesterolaemia and hypertriglyceridaemia have been reported during treatment with AP drugs as have modest increases in low-density lipoproteins and reductions in low-density lipoproteins. These changes are associated with weight gain and educational programmes that encourage appropriate diet, exercise and smoking cessation may be helpful.

Metabolic syndrome is at least twice as common in patients with schizophrenia as in controls. The metabolic adverse effects of AP drugs that have been discussed above have recently been reviewed in light of this (Thakore, 2005).

Cardiovascular adverse effects

Sudden cardiac death has long been reported in otherwise healthy young people, especially males, treated with AP drugs. The causes of such deaths may include:

* noradrenergic α_1 blockade, some AP drugs, especially in high dosage, causing marked blockade which may lead to profound hypotension
* concomitant treatment with drugs that act synergistically to cause cardiorespiratory collapse, for example benzodiazepine (BZD) drugs and
* intravenous (IV) administration or IM administration in overactive patients in whom skeletal muscle is so highly perfused with blood that IM administration is effectively the same as IV administration.

It has been recognised more recently that some sudden deaths may be caused by AP drugs blocking cardiac K^+ channels and causing prolongation of the QTc interval on the electrocardiogram. QTc prolongation may lead to ventricular tachyarrhythmias and death and is more likely to occur in patients who are hypokalaemic or have high sympathetic tone, both of which situations may prevail in agitated, overactive patients. The atypical AP drug sertindole has been reintroduced for use in the UK following an earlier suspension because of concerns about arrhythmias (see Table 8.4) and ziprasidone also carries this risk. Clozapine, olanzapine, quetiapine, amisulpride, aripiprazole, risperidone and zotepine appear to have no clinically significant effect on the QTc interval. Several typical AP drugs prolong the QTc interval and droperidol is no longer available while thioridazine is restricted to second-line treatment of schizophrenia in adults under specialist supervision.

Blood dyscrasias

Clozapine is associated with an increased risk of agranulocytosis and patients treated with it require haematological monitoring (both patients and prescribers must be registered with a clozapine monitoring service). Reversible neutropaenia occurs in 3% of clozapine-treated patients while 0.8% of patients developed agranulocytosis prior to the introduction of haematological monitoring.

Blood dyscrasias including leucopaenia and agranulocytosis have also been reported in patients treated with other atypical and typical AP drugs. All patients who are being treated with AP drugs and who develop unexplained infections or fevers should have full blood counts performed.

Elderly patients

AP drugs should be prescribed cautiously in elderly patients in whom the risk of dizziness and postural hypotension (which may lead to falls and hip fractures) is high. Elderly patients are also very susceptible to hyperthermia and hypothermia.

It has recently been recognised that atypical (and probably also typical) AP drugs increase the risk of both cerebrovascular events and mortality in elderly patients with dementia approximately threefold when compared with placebo. This has resulted in a somewhat confusing situation in which 'Dear Doctor Letters' (see Chapter 5) have been issued for olanzapine and risperidone and the CSM (2004) has advised that they should no longer be prescribed for disturbed behaviour in elderly patients with dementia, while a working group of the Royal College of Psychiatrists and others (2004) recommends the gradual withdrawal of olanzapine and risperidone in elderly patients with dementia but with the exception of those with a diagnosis of schizophrenia (who may have a history of cerebrovascular events) or who continue to have moderate to severe symptoms or to pose a risk of danger.

Specific adverse effects

The specific adverse effects of AP drugs may be attributed to their antagonist effect at DA D_2 neuroreceptors and are unlikely to be caused by other psychotropic drugs. They include EPS adverse effects and hyperprolactinaemia.

Extrapyramidal system adverse effects

EPS adverse effects were described before the invention of AP drugs but typical AP drugs greatly increase the risk for these disorders and atypical AP drugs are not without blame. These adverse effects are now briefly described.

- Acute dystonia consists of fixed contortions of the muscles of the head, neck and upper limbs. It occurs immediately or within a few days of treatment with an AP drug and is commonest in younger male patients. Acute dystonia responds rapidly to parenterally administered antimuscarinic drugs (see Chapter 15).

- Akathisia consists of distressing psychological restlessness and continuous movement that is not goal directed and that may resemble psychiatric disorder. It occurs equally in both sexes, particularly following high doses of AP drugs, and usually develops during the first few days or weeks of treatment. Antimuscarinic drugs have no effect on akathisia but benzodiazepine or beta-blocking drugs may be useful.

- Parkinsonism consists of the triad of bradykinesia, rigidity and tremor. It may only develop after some weeks of treatment and is commonest in older female patients. Parkinsonism may respond to lowering the dose of, or switching to an alternative, AP drug. Antimuscarinic drugs suppress Parkinsonism but should only be prescribed when it develops because they may increase risk for tardive dyskinesia (see Chapter 15).

- Tardive dyskinesia is a syndrome of abnormal involuntary movements, typically choreoathetoid and usually complex, rapid and stereotyped. Choreiform lip pursing, tongue protrusion and sucking and chewing movements occur in 80% of patients who develop it. Limbs are less often affected and trunk muscles and muscles of respiration rarely so. The incidence of tardive dyskinesia in patients treated with typical AP drugs is about 5% per year and the cumulative prevalence is between 20% and 25%. The incidence and cumulative prevalence in patients treated with atypical AP drugs is significantly lower at 1% and 5–10% respectively. It is commonest in older female patients.

- Neuroleptic malignant syndrome (NMS) consists of EPS symptoms (rigidity), fluctuating consciousness (delirium, stupor) and autonomic lability (hyperthermia, tachycardia, hypo- or hypertension, sweating, pallor, salivation and urinary incontinence). Severe NMS is relatively rare and most often develops within a few weeks of initiating or altering AP drug therapy. Marked elevation of creatinine phosphokinase occurs and aldolase, liver enzymes and white cells may also be raised. Thromboembolism and renal failure caused by myoglobinuria secondary to muscle necrosis are common. Untreated, death occurs from cardiovascular collapse, respiratory failure or secondary pneumonia in 10% to 20% of affected patients. NMS is a medical emergency that is best treated in an intensive care unit. AP therapy must be discontinued (and it will be appreciated that this is not immediately possible with depot AP drugs), the patient's temperature normalised, fluid and electrolyte balance restored and secondary infection treated. Diazepam, dantrolene or bromocriptine may be useful, as may amantadine and L-dopa. Recovered patients usually have no sequelae. Further AP treatment will often be necessary and should be with an AP drug from a different chemical group. Dosage should be increased extremely slowly and patients should be carefully monitored.

Hyperprolactinaemia

Hyperprolactinaemia, a side effect of all typical AP drugs, causes hypo-oestrogenaemia which in turn causes:

- galactorrhoea, amenorrhoea, altered ovarian function, loss of libido and an increased long-term risk for osteoporosis in women and
- gynaecomastia, impotence, loss of libido and impaired spermatogenesis in men.

Clozapine, olanzapine, quetiapine, aripiprazole and sertindole do not appear to be associated with significant hyperprolactinaemia, in contrast to both amisulpride and risperidone and to the typical AP drugs. The prolactin-sparing effect of these atypical AP drugs is almost certainly due to their low affinity for tuberoinfundibular D_2 receptors which allows DA to maintain its tonic control over prolactin secretion. Reducing risk for hyperprolactinaemia is highly desirable given that impotence in men and loss of libido in both sexes may impair the quality of patients' live and their adherence to treatment, while osteoporosis may present a longer-term personal and public health risk (Naidoo et al, 2003).

References and further reading

Bilder RM, Goldman RS, Volavka J et al (2002) Neurocognitive effects of clozapine, olanzapine, risperidone, and haloperidol in patients with chronic schizophrenia or schizoaffective disorder. American Journal of Psychiatry 159(6):1018–1028.

Chan CH, Janicak PG, Davis JM, Altman E, Andriukaitis S, Hedeker D (1987) Response of psychotic and nonpsychotic depressed patients to tricyclic antidepressants. Journal of Clinical Psychiatry 48(5):197–200.

Committee on Safety of Medicines (2004) Atypical antipsychotic drugs and stroke: Message from Professor Gordon Duff, Chairman, Committee on Safety of Medicines (CEM/CMO/2004/1) www.mca.gov.uk/aboutagency/regframework/csm/csmframe.htm (accessed May 2005).

Kapur S, Seeman P (2001) Does fast dissociation from the dopamine D_2 receptor explain the action of atypical antipsychotics?: A new hypothesis. American Journal of Psychiatry 158(3):360–369.

Kessler RM, Ansari MS, Riccardi P, Li R, Jayathilake K, Dawant B, Meltzer HY (2005) Occupancy of striatal and extrastriatal dopamine D(2)/D(3) receptors by olanzapine and haloperidol. Neuropsychopharmacology 30(12):2283–2289.

Lieberman JA, Tollefson GD, Charles C, et al for the HGDH Study Group (2005) Antipsychotic drug effects on brain morphology in first-episode psychosis. Archives of General Psychiatry 62(4):361–370.

Meltzer HY, Alphs L, Green AI, for the International Suicide Prevention Trial Study Group (2003) Clozapine treatment for suicidality in schizophrenia: International Suicide Prevention Trial (InterSePT). Archives of General Psychiatry 60(1):82–91.

Naidoo U, Goff DC, Klibanski A (2003) Hyperprolactinemia and bone mineral density: the potential impact of AP agents. Psychoneuroendocrinology Suppl. 2: 97–108.

National Institute for Clinical Excellence (2002) Schizophrenia: Core interventions in the treatment and management of schizophrenia in primary and secondary care. Online. Available at: www.nice.org.uk (accessed May 2005).

Pilowsky LS (2001) Probing targets for antipsychotic drug action with PET and SPET receptor imaging. Nucleic Medicine Communications 22(7):829–833.

Royal College of Psychiatrists (Faculty of the Psychiatry of Old Age, Royal College of General Practitioners and Alzheimer's Society). Summary – Guidance for the management of behavioural and psychiatric symptoms in dementia and the treatment of psychosis in people with history of stroke/TIA. www.rcpsych.ac.uk/college/faculty/oap/professional/guidance_summary.htm (accessed May 2005).

Thakore JH (2005) Metabolic syndrome and schizophrenia. British Journal of Psychiatry 186:455–456.

Tohen M, Greil W, Calabrese JR et al (2005) Olanzapine versus lithium in the maintenance treatment of bipolar disorder: a 12 month randomized double-blind controlled clinical trial. American Journal of Psychiatry 162(7):1281–1290.

World Health Organization (1973) Report of the International Pilot Study of Schizophrenia. Geneva: WHO.

Wright P, David S, Birkett M, et al (2003) Intramuscular olanzapine and intramuscular haloperidol in acute schizophrenia: antipsychotic efficacy and extrapyramidal safety during the first 24 hours of treatment. Canadian Journal of Psychiatry 48(11):647–652.

Wright P, O'Flaherty L (2003) Antipsychotic drugs: atypical advantages and typical disadvantages. Irish Journal of Psychological Medicine 20(1):24–27.

Zhang W, Bymaster FP (2000) In vivo receptor neurochemical studies with olanzapine. In: Olanzapine: A Novel Antipsychotic (Eds Tran PV, Bymaster FP, Tye N, et al). Philadelphia, Lippincott Williams and Wilkins, pp. 146–159.

9

Antidepressant drugs

Introduction

Any classification of the antidepressant (AD) drugs is unsatisfactory, whether it is based on their chemical structure, pharmacology or clinical effects. Therefore like the antipsychotic drugs, it is probably best to pragmatically divide them into two classes, the newer and the older AD drugs.

The newer AD drugs include:

- The selective serotonin (5HT) reuptake inhibitor (SSRI) AD drugs including citalopram and its isomer escitalopram, fluoxetine, fluvoxamine, paroxetine and sertraline.
- The 5HT and noradrenaline (NA; norepinephrine) reuptake inhibitor (SNRI) AD drugs venlafaxine and duloxetine.
- The reversible monoamine oxidase (MAO) Type A inhibitor AD drug moclobemide (sometimes referred to as a reversible inhibitor of MAO-A or RIMA) and
- A miscellaneous group that includes mirtazapine (a presynaptic NA α_2 and $5HT_{2A, 2C \& 3}$ receptor antagonist), reboxetine (a selective NA reuptake inhibitor) and tryptophan (the essential amino acid precursor of 5HT).

Bupropion (see below) is licensed as an adjuvant to cigarette smoking cessation in the UK, but is not licensed as an antidepressant (see Chapter 14).

The older AD drugs include:

- The tricyclic (TCA) AD drugs amitriptyline, amoxapine, clomipramine, dothiepin (now called dosulepin), doxepin, imipramine, lofepramine, nortriptyline and trimipramine (all of which are 5HT and NA reuptake inhibitors).
- The TCA-related AD drugs maprotiline (a tetracyclic selective NA reuptake inhibitor), mianserin (a tetracyclic and relatively selective NA reuptake inhibitor) and trazodone (a tetracyclic 5HT reuptake inhibitor and NA α_1 antagonist) and
- The MAO-A inhibitor (MAOI) AD drugs including isocarboxazid, phenelzine and tranylcypromine.

All of the AD drugs listed above may be regarded as first-line treatments for depression with the notable exception of the MAOI AD drugs. These interact with certain foods and with other drugs and are somewhat less effective than the other AD drugs. They are therefore generally reserved for treatment-resistant depression or atypical depression and treatment with them is usually only initiated by a psychiatrist.

Pharmacokinetics

It is convenient to consider the pharmacokinetics (PK) of the newer and older AD drugs separately.

Newer antidepressant drugs

Selective serotonin reuptake inhibitors

All of the SSRI AD drugs – citalopram, escitalopram, fluoxetine, fluvoxamine, paroxetine and sertraline – are slowly but completely absorbed from the proximal small intestine and reach C_{MAX} in 4–8 hours. They are subject to extensive first pass metabolism and several active metabolites are produced, for example norfluoxetine in the case of fluoxetine (see below). Protein binding exceeds 90% for most SSRI AD drugs but is approximately 75% for citalopram and fluvoxamine. The $T_{1/2}$ of most SSRI AD drugs is <12 hours but is considerably longer for fluoxetine at 72 hours. SSRI discontinuation symptoms occur with reducing frequency as $T_{1/2}$ increases (see below).

Serotonin and noradrenaline (norepinephrine) reuptake inhibitors

The SNRI venlafaxine is readily absorbed from the proximal small intestine and reaches C_{MAX} in 3 hours. It is subject to extensive first pass metabolism which produces the active metabolite O-desmethylvenlafaxine. Plasma protein binding is low at approximately 25%. The $T_{1/2}$ of venlafaxine is approximately 5 hours.

Duloxetine is administered as a single enantiomer (see Chapter 4) and is readily absorbed, reaching C_{MAX} in 6 hours. It is subject to extensive first pass metabolism but has no active metabolites. Plasma protein binding is approximately 95%. The $T_{1/2}$ of duloxetine is approximately 12 hours.

Reversible monoamine oxidase type A inhibitors

The MAO-A inhibitor or RIMA, moclobemide, is readily and completely absorbed from the proximal small intestine reaching C_{MAX} in 1 hour. It is subject to extensive first pass metabolism which produces metabolites that are almost completely inactive. Plasma protein binding is approximately 50%. The $T_{1/2}$ of moclobemide is approximately 3 hours.

Miscellaneous newer antidepressant drugs

The miscellaneous group of newer AD drugs includes mirtazapine, reboxetine and tryptophan. Mirtazapine is readily absorbed from the proximal small intestine and reaches C_{MAX} in 2 hours. It is subject to extensive first pass metabolism which produces the active metabolite demethyl mirtazapine. Plasma protein binding is approximately 85%. It is has a $T_{1/2}$ of approximately 30 hours.

Reboxetine is readily absorbed and reaches C_{MAX} in 2 hours. Plasma protein binding is extensive at 97% and it has a $T_{1/2}$ of approximately 12 hours.

L-tryptophan, an essential amino acid, is readily absorbed and reaches C_{MAX} in 2 hours. Plasma protein binding is extensive.

Older antidepressant drugs

Tricyclic antidepressant drugs

The TCA AD drugs amitriptyline, amoxapine, clomipramine, dothiepin (dosulepin), doxepin, imipramine, lofepramine, nortriptyline and trimipramine have relatively similar PK. Thus:

- Absorption is rapid and almost complete at the proximal small intestine and C_{MAX} is reached in from 2 (for tertiary amines such as amitriptyline and imipramine) to 6 (for secondary amines such as nortriptyline) hours.
- They are subject to extensive first pass metabolism by hydroxylation and demethylation and only 50% of absorbed drug appears in the systemic circulation. Most TCA AD drugs have active metabolites. Alcohol increases first pass metabolism of TCA AD drugs (by enzyme induction)

in those who consume it regularly but reduces it (by competition for enzyme) in those who consume it infrequently. This probably accounts for some of the mortality associated with overdoses involving both TCA AD drugs and alcohol.

* Plasma protein binding is up to 95%.
* $T_{1/2}$ is approximately 24 hours.
* They are eliminated via the kidney.

Tricyclic-related antidepressant drugs

The TCA-related AD drugs maprotiline, mianserin and trazodone are completely absorbed. They are extensively metabolised with the production of active metabolites. Plasma protein binding is 90% and $T_{1/2}$ is approximately 8 hours.

Monoamine oxidase inhibitors

MAO A and B in presynaptic mitochondria catalyse the oxidative deamination of 5HT, NA and, to a lesser extent, dopamine (DA), following their reuptake by transporter proteins on the presynaptic membrane. The MAOI AD drugs isocarboxazid, phenelzine and tranylcypromine are transformed by MAO into products that irreversibly inactivate MAO, thus increasing synaptic neuro-transmitter concentrations (Fig. 9.1). The effect of an MAOI therefore persists for up to two weeks after treatment with it has been discontinued and is only reversed following synthesis of new enzyme.

Isocarboxazid, tranylcypromine and phenelzine all irreversibly inactivate MAO A which preferentially degrades NA and 5HT. Isocarboxazid and tranylcypromine irreversibly inactivate MAO B which degrades NA, 5HT and DA. Tranylcypromine has a structure similar to that of amfetamine (see Chapter 7) and may also have a central stimulant action.

MOA B also catalyses the oxidative deamination of neuroprotoxins to neurotoxins. Neurotoxins are implicated in neurodegenerative disorders such as Parkinson's disease. Selegeline, a selective and irreversible MAO B inhibitor, may be beneficial to patients with Parkinson's disease.

Pharmacodynamics

The mechanism of action of AD drugs appears to depend on their ability to increase synaptic concentrations of some or all of the biogenic amines 5HT, NA and DA. The mechanisms by which AD drugs increase synaptic concentrations of biogenic amines are discussed further below but briefly include:

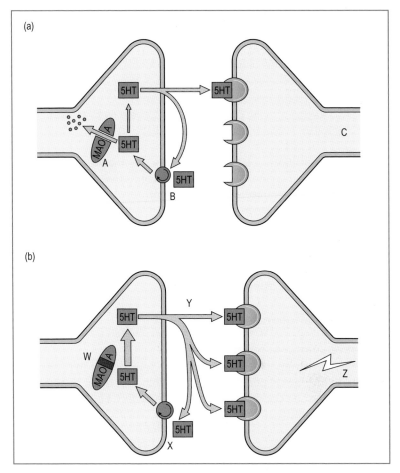

Fig. 9.1 Mechanism of action of monoamine oxidase inhibitor antidepressant drugs in the treatment of depression. (**a**) MAO A in the presynaptic mitochondria (A) catalyses the oxidative deamination of 5HT (and also NA and DA) following its reuptake by transporter proteins (B). This reduces the amount of 5HT available for release into the synapse and inhibits neurotransmission and depolarisation of the postsynaptic neurone (C). (**b**) MAOI antidepressant drugs are transformed (by MAO itself) into products that irreversibly inactivate MAO (W). This prevents oxidative deamination of 5HT following its reuptake by transporter proteins (X) and increases the amount of 5HT available for release into the synapse (Y). This in turn facilitates neurotransmission and depolarisation of the postsynaptic neurone (Z).

- Inhibition of the transporter proteins on the presynaptic membrane responsible for the reuptake of 5HT, NA and DA from the synapse to the presynaptic neurone.
- Inhibition of MAO, the degradative enzyme for 5HT, NA and DA, in the presynaptic mitochondria of the terminal axon fibres.
- Blockade of presynaptic 5HT and NA neuroreceptors which prevents negative feedback to the presynaptic neurone and thus permits further synthesis and release into the synapse of 5HT and NA.

These three effects of AD drugs may be regarded as primary mechanisms of action in that they in turn have further, secondary effects on postsynaptic neurones and on other neuronal systems that these neurones modulate. Increased synaptic concentrations of biogenic amines cause increased expression of several genes in the nuclei of postsynaptic neurones, for example, while increased synaptic 5HT concentrations cause downregulation of postsynaptic $5HT_2$ neuroreceptors.

As with PK, it is convenient to consider the pharmacodynamics of the newer and older AD drugs separately.

Newer antidepressant drugs

Selective serotonin reuptake inhibitors

The SSRI AD drugs selectively block the reuptake of 5HT from the synapse to the presynaptic neurone via inhibition of the 5HT transporter protein located on the presynaptic membrane (see Fig. 9.2). They also weakly inhibit the reuptake of NA from the synapse to the presynaptic neurone via inhibition of the NA transporter protein.

Older AD drugs, particularly clomipramine, have a similar mechanism of action to the SSRI AD drugs but unlike them they are also potent antagonists at postsynaptic NA α_1, histaminergic H_1 and cholinergic (Ach) muscarinic M_1 neuroreceptors (see below).

Serotonin and noradrenaline (norepinephrine) reuptake inhibitors

The measurement of the affinity of psychotopic drugs for neuro-receptors *in vivo* has been described in Chapter 8 and it will be recalled that the lower the K_i, the greater the affinity of the drug for the receptor. Venlafaxine potently inhibits the reuptake of both 5HT and NA from the synapse to the presynaptic neurone via their presynaptic transporter proteins. This inhibition of binding has been quantified as 82 and 2483 Ki nM for the 5HT and NA transporter proteins respectively (Wong and Bymaster, 2002). The differential affinity of venlafaxine for the 5HT and NA transporter proteins means that its mechanism of action changes from that of an SSRI at low dose (<150 mg daily) to that of an SNRI at higher dose (>150 mg daily).

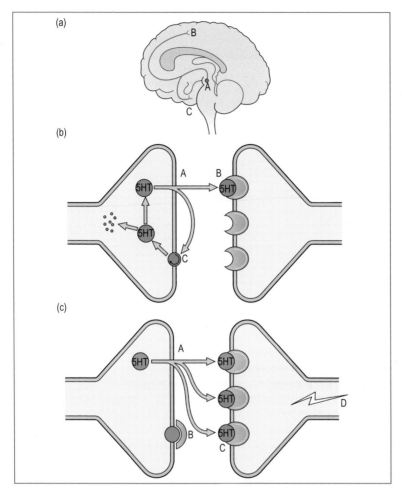

Fig. 9.2 Mechanism of action of selective serotonin reuptake inhibitor antidepressant drugs. (**a**) SSRI AD drugs promote the activity of serotonergic neurones that originate in the raphe nuclei (A) and project to cortex (B) and limbic system (C). AD drugs such as reboxetine, nortriptyline, maprotiline and mianserin promote the activity of noradrenergic neurones that originate in the locus ceruleus and project to cortex and limbic system while TCA AD drugs promote the activity of both serotonergic and noradrenergic systems (see also Fig. 3.4). (**b**) Serotonin (5HT) is released from the presynaptic neurone (A) and either binds to postsynaptic 5HT receptors (B) or re-enters the presynaptic neurone via the reuptake transporter protein (C) located on the presynaptic membrane. (**c**) SSRI AD drugs have no effect on 5HT release from the presynaptic neurone (A) but they selectively block the reuptake of 5HT from the synapse to the presynaptic neurone via inhibition of the 5HT transporter protein (B). This increases synaptic 5HT concentration, promotes 5HT binding to postsynaptic receptors (C) and facilitates neuronal firing (D). AD drugs such as reboxetine, nortriptyline, maprotiline and mianserin have a similar mechanism of action at the NA transporter protein while TCA AD drugs have this effect at both 5HT and NA transporter proteins.

Table 9.1: Inhibition of binding to human monoamine reuptake transporter proteins (Ki, nM) by representative antidepressant drugs (Wong and Bymaster, 2002)

Class	Drug	5HT transporter protein	NA transporter protein
SSRI	Citalopram	1.2	4070
	Fluoxetine	0.8	240
	Fluvoxamine	2.2	1300
	Paroxetine	0.1	40
	Sertraline	0.3	420
SNRI	Venlafaxine	82	2480
	Duloxetine	0.8	7.5
TCA	Clomipramine	0.3	38

Duloxetine is an even more potent inhibitor than venlafaxine of the reuptake of both 5HT and NA from the synapse to the presynaptic neurone via their presynaptic transporter proteins. Its inhibition of binding to NA and 5HT transporter molecules has been quantified as 7.5 and 0.8 Ki nM respectively (Wong and Bymaster, 2002).

Older AD drugs including the TCA and TCA-related AD drugs have a similar mechanism of action to the SNRI AD drugs but unlike them they are also potent antagonists at postsynaptic NA α_1, histaminergic H_1 and Ach muscarinic M_1 neuroreceptors (see below).

Reversible monoamine oxidase type A inhibitors

MAO-A and MAO-B are located in the presynaptic mitochondria where they catalyse the oxidative deamination of 5HT, NA and, to a lesser extent, DA, following their reuptake by transporter proteins. The RIMA, moclobemide, reversibly and selectively inhibits MAO-A thus increasing presynaptic neuronal, and subsequently synaptic, concentrations of these biogenic amines.

Miscellaneous newer antidepressant drugs

Mirtazapine prevents synaptic neurotransmitters from exerting negative feedback on the presynaptic neurone by blocking presynaptic autoreceptors (see Chapter 3). The presynaptic neurone therefore continues to synthesise neurotransmitter and to release it into the synapse. This increases synaptic concentrations of both 5HT and NA. It is thought that the S enantiomer of mirtazepine blocks NA α_2 and

$5HT_{2A \& 2C}$ receptors while the R enantiomer blocks $5HT_3$ receptors. Mirtazapine's sedative action is thought to be mediated via blockade of histamine H_1 receptors.

Reboxetine is a selective NA reuptake inhibitor that has no appreciable effect on 5HT or DA. This has led to the suggestion that it might be best employed in combination therapy with an SSRI or RIMA.

L-tryptophan, an essential amino acid, is converted to 5HT by hydroxylation and decarboxylation. It is believed that brain concentrations of 5HT are low in depression and that oral administration of L-tryptophan restores them to normal.

Older antidepressant drugs

Tricyclic antidepressant drugs

TCA AD drugs inhibit the reuptake of both 5HT and NA (and DA to a much lesser extent) via their transporter proteins to the presynaptic neurone. This increases synaptic concentrations of these biogenic amines and thus enhances neurotransmission. The secondary amines desipramine and nortriptyline inhibit NA reuptake to a much greater extent than 5HT reuptake while clomipramine has the opposite effect. Biogenic amine reuptake inhibition occurs within hours of taking TCA AD drugs but their antidepressant effect may not become evident for several weeks. It is thought that this is because while biogenic amine reuptake inhibition is necessary for the antidepressant effect of TCA AD drugs, it is not sufficient. In addition, adaptive changes in pre- and postsynaptic neuroreceptors in response to stimulation by increased concentrations of biogenic amines are thought to be further necessary steps that occur more gradually. Such adaptive changes include:

- upregulation of presynaptic NA α_1 receptors
- downregulation of postsynaptic NA α_2 receptors and
- increased expression of genes coding for brain-derived neurotrophic factor and other proteins.

TCA AD drugs also bind to postsynaptic neuroreceptors including NA α_1, histamine H_1, Ach and muscarinic M_1 neuroreceptors. This binding is thought to mediate their adverse effects (see below).

Tricyclic-related antidepressant drugs

The tetracyclic AD drug maprotiline is a selective NA reuptake inhibitor that has no appreciable effect on 5HT or DA. It has slight affinity for postsynaptic NA α_1, and marked affinity for histaminergic H_1 and Ach muscarinic M_1 neuroreceptors.

Mianserin prevents synaptic neurotransmitters from exerting negative feedback on the presynaptic neurone by blocking presynaptic NA α_2 and 5HT autoreceptors (see Chapter 3). The presynaptic neurone therefore continues to synthesise neurotransmitter and to release it into the synapse. This increases synaptic concentrations of both 5HT and NA.

The mechanism of action of the triazolopyridine trazodone (and of nefazadone, which is no longer available in the UK) is poorly understood. It does not inhibit NA reuptake via the transporter protein but is thought to be an antagonist at central $5HT_2$ receptors.

Monoamine oxidase inhibitor drugs

MAO A and B in presynaptic mitochondria catalyse the oxidative deamination of 5HT, NA and, to a lesser extent, DA, following their reuptake by transporter proteins. The MAOI AD drugs isocarboxazid, phenelzine and tranylcypromine are transformed by MAO into products that irreversibly inactivate MAO, thus increasing synaptic neurotransmitter concentrations. The effect of an MAOI therefore persists for up to two weeks after treatment with it has been discontinued and is only reversed following synthesis of new enzyme.

Isocarboxazid, tranylcypromine and phenelzine all irreversibly inactivate MAO A which preferentially degrades NA and 5HT. Isocarboxazid and tranylcypromine irreversibly inactivate MAO B which degrades NA, 5HT and DA. Tranylcypromine has a structure similar to that of amfetamine (see Chapter 7) and may also have a central stimulant action.

Psychopharmacology and our understanding of depression

An understanding of the mechanism of action of AD drugs has contributed significantly to our knowledge of the pathophysiology of depression. It has also contributed to our understanding of anxiety disorders (see Chapter 11).

The monoamine hypothesis of depression

The monoamine hypothesis of depression was proposed soon after the TCA and MAOI AD drugs were invented and following the discovery that they both increased synaptic concentrations of biogenic amines. It states that depression is caused by reduced synaptic concentrations of 5HT, NA and DA and/or their postsynaptic receptors. It is supported by the following observations:

- All AD drugs increase synaptic concentrations of some or all of the biogenic amines 5HT, NA and DA.

- Reserpine causes depletion of biogenic amines and leads to depression.
- Concentrations of the biogenic amine metabolites 5-hydroxyindolacetic acid (HIAA), homovanillic acid (HVA) and 3 methoxy 4 hydroxy phenylglycol (MHPG) are reduced in cerebrospinal fluid from depressed patients.

The monoamine hypothesis raised the question of whether one or other of 5HT, NA and DA was primarily implicated in depression. Attempts to answer this question produced specific serotonergic, noradrenergic and other hypotheses.

The serotonergic hypothesis of depression

The 5HT hypothesis was proposed by Coppen (1967) and has been reviewed by Maes and Meltzer (1997). It is supported by the following observations (for review see Cleare, 2005):

- The SSRI AD drugs alleviate depression by selectively increasing synaptic concentrations of 5HT while having no significant effect on synaptic concentrations of NA or DA.
- Neuroendocrine challenge paradigms point to impaired 5HT neurotransmission in depressed patients. The 5HT-mediated increase in prolactin secretion that occurs in healthy individuals in response to D-fenfluramine, for example, is blunted in depressed patients and normalises following successful treatment.
- The concentration of tryptophan is reduced in plasma from depressed patients suggesting impaired uptake of this 5HT precursor.
- The concentration of 5HT is reduced in platelets from depressed patients.
- MAOI AD drugs administered concomitantly with tryptophan are more effective in treating depression than MAOI monotherapy.
- Functional neuroimaging provides some evidence of reduced $5HT_{1A}$ and $5HT_2$ binding in the brains of depressed patients. Curiously perhaps, this does not appear to normalise following successful treatment.
- Perhaps the strongest evidence of a causal link between impaired 5HT neurotransmission and depression comes from the tryptophan depletion paradigm.

Experimental tryptophan depletion

Tryptophan is an essential amino acid precursor of 5HT that raises synaptic 5HT concentrations simply by providing more substrate for conversion to 5HT. Experimental tryptophan depletion may be accomplished by a diet that provides an excess intake of neutral amino acids which saturate the brain's amino acid transporter and prevent tryptophan uptake to the brain. This causes rapid and marked lowering of mood with prominent psychomotor retardation in depressed patients who have been successfully treated with AD drugs acting on 5HT systems such as SSRI AD drugs. This effect is not evident in similar patients treated successfully with AD drugs acting on NA systems, for example the secondary amine TCA AD drugs desipramine and nortriptyline (Delgado et al, 1999).

The noradrenergic hypothesis of depression

The NA hypothesis is supported by the following observations:

- The AD drugs reboxetine, nortriptyline, maprotiline and mianserin alleviate depression by selectively increasing synaptic concentrations of NA while having little effect on synaptic concentrations of 5HT or DA.
- Neuroendocrine challenge paradigms point to impaired NA neurotransmission in depressed patients. The NA-mediated increase in growth hormone secretion that occurs in healthy individuals in response to desipramine, for example, is blunted in depressed patients.
- The experimental NA depletion paradigm.

Experimental noradrenaline (norepinephrine) depletion

Experimental NA depletion may be accomplished by treatment with α methyl paratyrosine which inhibits tyrosine hydroxylase, the enzyme that catalyses the conversion of tyrosine to DOPA (or dihydroxyphenylalanine) and thence to DA and NA. This causes marked lowering of mood in depressed patients who have been successfully treated with AD drugs acting on NA systems such as TCA AD drugs. This effect is not evident in similar patients treated successfully with AD drugs acting on 5HT systems, for example SSRI AD drugs.

Other hypotheses of depression

A DA hypothesis of depression has been proposed because:

- bupropion, an effective AD drug, is a selective DA and NA reuptake inhibitor that has little effect on the reuptake of 5HT and does not inhibit MAO (although its precise mechanism of action is not well understood) and
- neuroendocrine challenge paradigms point to impaired DA neurotransmission in depressed patients. The DA-mediated increase in growth hormone secretion that occurs in healthy individuals in response to apomorphine, for example, is blunted in depressed patients.

Cholinergic and gamma-amino butyrate-ergic theories have also been proposed as has a monoamine interaction theory. These and the effects of AD drugs on gene expression in neurones, currently an area of intense research, are beyond the scope of this volume but are well described by Cleare (2005) as are neuroendocrine and monoamine/neuroendocrine interaction hypotheses.

Efficacy

AD drugs are effective in:

- treating major depressive disorder (MDD) and similar syndromes (depression with anxiety, depression with psychotic symptoms, atypical depression, dysthymia and premenstrual dysphoric disorder)
- preventing new episodes of depression in patients who have been successfully treated for MDD and similar syndromes
- treating depressive relapse in patients with bipolar disorder (bipolar depression)
- treating anxiety disorders including obsessive compulsive disorder, panic disorder, post-traumatic stress disorder, generalised anxiety disorder and social phobia (see Chapter 11)
- treating bulimia nervosa
- treating chronic pain syndromes including diabetic neuropathy and postherpetic neuralgia (SNRI and TCA AD drugs but not SSRI AD drugs)
- treating nocturnal enuresis in children (see Chapter 7) and
- treating premature ejaculation (SSRI AD drugs) (see Chapter 13).

Major depressive disorder

When compared with the older AD drugs, the main advantage of the newer AD drugs is their safety. They cause fewer adverse effects and thus patients may be more willing to take them, and they are significantly safer in overdose (see below).

There is no unequivocal evidence that newer AD drugs are more effective than the older AD drugs in treating MDD although venlafaxine and duloxetine may be exceptions in this regard. However, treatment with many newer AD drugs may be initiated at the therapeutic dose, a factor which shortens time to recovery and precludes sub-therapeutic dosing.

It therefore seems appropriate on the grounds of safety and appropriateness of dose to recommend newer AD drugs as the first-line medication for the vast majority of patients who require such treatment and especially for:

- patients with histories of intolerance to older AD drugs and/or of poor adherence to treatment
- patients with histories of overdosing, particularly with older AD drugs
- patients with general medical disorders, particularly cardiovascular disorders, and
- patients taking concomitant medications.

The National Institute for Clinical Excellence (NICE) has recommended that when an AD drug is to be prescribed in routine care, it should be an SSRI because these are as effective as TCA AD drugs but are less likely to be discontinued because of adverse effects (2004).

Individual older AD drugs may be appropriate for some patients, for example patients who have responded to them previously. It is worth noting that several newer AD drugs are now available generically and thus cost should not be a factor in determining treatment.

All patients for whom AD drugs are to be prescribed must be informed about their efficacy and adverse effects and about the anticipated duration of treatment (see Box 9.1).

Acute treatment

Treatment of MDD should commence with an adequate dose of a single newer AD drug. If this proves ineffective after 2–3 weeks the dose should be increased and treatment continued for a further 2–3 weeks. If treatment remains ineffective this drug should be discontinued, a second newer AD drug should be prescribed and the same two-stage process should be repeated. If the second drug proves ineffective the treatment strategies described below for treatment-resistant depression should be considered. The importance of treatment with an adequate dose of a newer AD drug for an adequate duration of time cannot be overemphasised.

If the first newer AD drug prescribed is not tolerated the patient should be switched to treatment with a second newer AD drug. If this is not tolerated the treatment strategies described below for treatment-resistant depression should be considered.

A combination of AD and antipsychotic (AP) drugs should be prescribed for patients with MDD who are experiencing psychotic symptoms.

Box 9.1: Information that must be provided to patients for whom antidepressant drugs are to be prescribed

nice guidelines

- The antidepressant effect of AD drugs does not occur immediately and may take several weeks to become evident.
- Any individual drug may not be effective and it may be necessary to try 2 or 3 different AD drugs until one is found which is effective (patients who have responded to any individual AD drug when previously depressed are likely to respond to it again if a further episode of MDD occurs).
- Dose-related adverse effects (see below) are commonly experienced by patients taking SSRI and SNRI AD drugs during the first week of treatment but these usually resolve with continued treatment.
- If effective, AD drugs need to be continued for 6–12 months following full recovery in order to prevent relapse (for patients with recurrent depression it may be appropriate to advise that treatment may need to be continued indefinitely).
- Craving, tolerance and addiction do not occur.
- A discontinuation syndrome (see below) may occur if doses of AD drug are omitted or it treatment is discontinued abruptly, particularly in the case of paroxetine and venlafaxine.
- Persistent adverse effects (see below) may develop with continued treatment but these can usually be ameliorated.
- Discontinuing treatment with AD drugs should be undertaken gradually by tapering the dose over several weeks or months.

MAOI AD drugs should be reserved for second-line management of treatment-resistant depression and for atypical depression. Their use should only be initiated by a psychiatrist and patients taking them should be monitored by a clinician familiar with their benefits and adverse effects.

The following rules should be observed when switching patients from one class of AD drug to another:

- An interval of 1 week (5 weeks in the case of fluoxetine) should elapse between discontinuing treatment with an SSRI and commencing treatment with an MAOI.
- An interval of 2 weeks should elapse between discontinuing treatment with a TCA and commencing treatment with an MAOI.
- An interval of 2 weeks should elapse between discontinuing treatment with an MAOI and commencing treatment with either an SSRI, a TCA or another MAOI.

The starting dose, dose range and available formulations of the AD drugs currently licensed in the UK are presented in Table 9.2.

Maintenance treatment

Patients who respond to AD drug therapy and then discontinue treatment have a high risk of relapse, especially during the first 12 months following full recovery (Geddes et al, 2003). The majority of such patients should continue to take the AD drug that they responded to ('the AD drug that gets you well is the AD drug that keeps you well') at the same dosage ('the dose that gets you well is the dose that keeps you well') for at least 6 months and ideally for 12 months following full recovery. NICE has recommended that patients who have had two or more depressive episodes in the recent past, and who have experienced significant functional impairment during these episodes, should be advised to continue AD drugs for 2 years (2004). Indeed such prophylactic treatment may need to be continued for several years and sometimes indefinitely in patients with recurrent depressive disorder.

The eventual discontinuation of prophylactic AD drug therapy should be tapered over a minimum of 6–8 weeks in order to prevent the occurrence of discontinuation syndrome (see below).

Major depressive disorder in children and adolescents

The general advice provided above is applicable when AD drugs are prescribed for children suffering with depression. However, it is important to note that there is no SSRI or SNRI AD drug licensed in the UK for the treatment of MDD in patients <18 years old. The CSM issued advice to clinicians about the use of such AD drugs in this population in 2003 and updated this more recently (2005). The CSM advise that the benefit/risk balance for the treatment of depressive illness in patients <18 years old:

- is favourable for fluoxetine (which is licensed for the treatment of depression in paediatric patients in the US)
- cannot be assessed for fluvoxamine and
- is unfavourable for citalopram, escitalopram, mirtazapine, paroxetine, sertraline and venlafaxine.

Bipolar depressive episode (bipolar depression)

Although manic episode is essential to the diagnosis of bipolar disorder, depression is the dominant pathological mood that patients

Table 9.2: The initial daily dose, daily dose range and available formulations of the AD drugs that are currently approved in the UK

	AD drug	Initial dose[1]	Dose range[1]	Available formulations
Newer AD drugs	SSRI			
	Citalopram	10–20 mg	20–60 mg	Tablets Liquid
	Escitalopram	10 mg	10–20 mg	Tablets
	Fluoxetine	20 mg	20–60 mg	Capsules Liquid
	Fluvoxamine	50–100 mg	100–300 mg	Tablets
	Paroxetine[2]	20 mg	20–50 mg	Tablets Liquid
	Sertraline	50 mg	50–200 mg	Tablets
	SNRI			
	Duloxetine	60 mg	30–120 mg	Capsules
	Venlafaxine[3]	75 mg	75–375 mg	Tablets Capsules
	RIMA			
	Moclobemide	300 mg	150–600 mg	Tablets

(cont'd)

Table 9.2: The initial daily dose, daily dose range and available formulations of the AD drugs that are currently approved in the UK—cont'd

		AD drug	Initial dose[1]	Dose range[1]	Available formulations
Newer AD drugs	Miscellaneous	Mirtazapine	15 mg	15–45 mg	Tablets Orodispersible tablets Liquid
		Reboxetine	8 mg	8–12 mg	Tablets
		Tryptophan[4]	3 grams	3–6 grams	Tablets
Older AD drugs	TCA	Amitriptyline	75 mg	50–150 mg	Tablets Liquid
		Amoxapine	100–150 mg	150–300 mg	Tablets
		Clomipramine	10 mg	30–250 mg	Tablets Capsules
		Dothiepin (dosulepin)	75 mg	150–225 mg	Tablets Capsules
		Doxepin	75 mg	75–300 mg	Capsules
		Imipramine	75 mg	150–300 mg	Tablets
		Lofepramine	140–210 mg	140–210 mg	Tablets Liquid

Table 9.2: The initial daily dose, daily dose range and available formulations of the AD drugs that are currently approved in the UK—cont'd

	AD drug	Initial dose[1]	Dose range[1]	Available formulations
Older AD drugs	Nortriptyline	75–100 mg	75–150 mg	Tablets
	Trimipramine	50–75 mg	150–300 mg	Tablets Capsules
TCA related	Maprotiline	25–75 mg	75–150 mg	Tablets
	Mianserin	30–40 mg	30–90 mg	Tablets
	Trazodone	150 mg	150–600 mg	Tablets Capsules Liquid
MAOI	Isocarboxazid	30 mg	30–60 mg	Tablets
	Phenelzine	45 mg	45–90 mg	Tablets
	Tranylcypromine	20 mg	20–30 mg	Tablets

Notes:

[1]The above dosing recommendations refer only to the treatment of MDD and dosing recommendations may differ when the AD drugs listed are used in the treatment of anxiety disorders or eating disorders (see below and Chapter 11).

[2]The Committee on Safety of Medicines (CSM) recommend 20 mg as the daily dose of paroxetine in the treatment of major depressive disorder, social phobia, generalised anxiety disorder and post-traumatic stress disorder and 40 mg as the daily dose of paroxetine in the treatment of obsessive-compulsive disorder and panic disorder on grounds that there is no evidence that higher doses are more effective (see text).

[3]The CSM recommend that treatment with venlafaxine should be initiated and monitored by a specialist (including general practitioners with experience in psychiatry) because of concerns about cardiotoxicity and toxicity in overdose.

[4]Prescribers and patients must be registered with the Optimax Information and Clinical Support unit (OPTICS) before treatment with tryptophan may be commenced.

with this disorder experience. Thus one study found that such patients were depressed 32%, manic or hypomanic 9% and either rapid cycling or experiencing mixed episodes 6% of the time over a mean period of 12.8 years (Judd et al, 2002). Furthermore up to 50% of patients with bipolar disorder attempt suicide at least once while approximately 15% die by suicide (Kessler et al, 1994; Jamison, 2000).

Bipolar depressive episode is usually referred to as bipolar depression. Its treatment is complex and combination therapy with AD, AP and mood stabilising drugs is widely employed. However:

- AD monotherapy may induce manic episodes, a risk that has been quantified as 3.7% with SSRI and 11.2% with TCA AD drugs, compared with 4.2% with placebo (Peet, 1994).
- AP and mood stabilising drugs may worsen depression.
- The optimal duration of AD therapy following response is not established although there is evidence that shorter durations are associated with earlier relapse (Altschuler et al, 2003).
- Mood stabilising drugs are more effective in preventing manic rather than depressive relapse.

Patients with bipolar depression should be treated with an SSRI AD drug and, in most cases, a concomitantly administered mood stabilising drug such as lithium, valproate or olanzapine (see Chapter 10). The choice of AD and mood stabilising drug should be guided, when possible, by the patient's previous response to such treatments. Otherwise lithium may be best for patients who experience manic and depressive relapse equally while olanzapine may be appropriate for those who experience predominantly manic relapse, and lamotrigine for those who experience predominantly depressive relapse.

Detailed advice on the treatment of bipolar disorder including bipolar depression is now available from a number of committees and consensus groups (for review see Fountoulakis et al, 2005) and draft NICE guidance is available with final guidance expected in June 2006.

Given that MDD and bipolar depression warrant different treatment regimens, the importance of detecting historical hypomanic or manic episodes which did not come to medical attention contemporaneously in patients presenting with a current episode of depression will be appreciated.

Treatment-resistant depression

Treatment-resistant depression may be defined as failure to respond to two different newer AD drugs prescribed in adequate doses for an adequate duration of time. Some experts would refine this definition by requiring that the two AD drugs be from two different AD drug classes, e.g. an SSRI and an SNRI AD drug.

The management of treatment-resistant depression is not as well defined as that of treatment-resistant schizophrenia. However, a number of strategies are available as follows:

- Review the diagnosis and consider the possibility of misdiagnosis and/or comorbidity, especially the presence of a general medical disorder such as hypothyroidism or occult neoplasm.
- Review the apparently ineffective treatment and consider the possibility of non-compliance with treatment, inadequate dosage or inadequate duration of treatment.
- Prescribe a drug from a different AD class (including MAOI) or prescribe venlafaxine or duloxetine if not already tried.
- Consider dual drug therapy with either an AD drug and an atypical AP drug, an AD drug and lithium, an AD drug and tryptophan or two AD drugs from two different classes (TCA with SSRI or TCA with MAOI). SSRIs, clomipramine and venlafaxine should not be combined with MAOIs because of the risk of 'serotonin syndrome' (see below).
- Consider triple drug therapy with an AD drug, lithium and tryptophan.
- Consider the addition of thyroxine (as liothyronine) to one of the above strategies.

Electroconvulsive therapy (ECT) would generally be considered before triple drug therapy or the addition of thyroxine and many psychiatrists would consider ECT if treatment with two different newer AD drugs prescribed in adequate doses for an adequate duration of time proves ineffective. ECT is recommended at an earlier stage if a patient's physical health or life is endangered (see Chapter 17). Tryptophan is available in the UK for prescription by hospital-based psychiatrists in combination with other AD drugs for patients who have been depressed for at least 2 years and who have not responded to AD monotherapy. Both patients and prescribers must register with OPTICS, the tryptophan monitoring service (see Table 9.2 and below).

Safety

AD drugs primarily modify 5HT- and NA-mediated neurotransmission but they also exert an effect at many other central and peripheral receptors as described above. These latter effects are, in the main, regarded as being responsible for the adverse effects of AD drugs although the precise causes of many adverse effects are unknown.

Newer antidepressant drugs

A discussion of two adverse effects that have been associated specifically with the newer AD drugs as a class – increased suicidal behaviour and discontinuation syndrome – will be followed by commentaries on the adverse effects associated with each of the different classes of newer AD drugs.

Increased suicidal behaviour

It is generally accepted that depressed patients are at increased risk of suicidal thoughts, self-harm and suicide and that the risk of these experiences is greatest when such patients first present for treatment and during the initial phase of their treatment.

Data available from a large number of research studies led the CSM to conclude in 2005 that a modest increase in the risk of suicidal thoughts and self harm for SSRI AD drugs compared with placebo cannot be excluded and is greatest for patients <18 years old. The CSM have therefore advised that all patients should be carefully monitored when treatment with SSRI AD drugs is initiated or dosages altered and that the benefit/risk balance for the treatment of depressive illness in patients <18 years old is favourable only for fluoxetine (see above).

The US Food and Drug Administration has also reviewed the available data and concluded that 4% of SSRI-treated patients experience suicidal thoughts and self-harm compared with 2% of placebo-treated patients. The FDA has issued advice that is similar to that of the CSM and has noted that only fluoxetine is approved for paediatric use in the US.

Discontinuation syndrome

A discontinuation syndrome occurs in 1 in 3 patients within 24 hours of abruptly discontinuing treatment with SSRI AD drugs. The symptoms may be moderate or severe and include anxiety, mood disturbance, gastrointestinal disturbance, dizziness, paraesthesia, sleep disturbance and an influenza-like syndrome of headache, arthralgia, myalgia, coryza, sweating and rigors. Discontinuation syndrome presents a problem to patients because a proportion are significantly disabled by it, and to clinicians because some of its symptoms – mood, gastrointestinal and sleep disturbance – may lead to the mistaken diagnosis of depressive relapse.

SSRI discontinuation syndrome is most common with paroxetine which has a short $T_{1/2}$ and is very uncommon with fluoxetine which has a long $T_{1/2}$ and an active major metabolite (norfluoxetine) which itself has a very long $T_{1/2}$ (2 weeks). It is also commonly experienced with venlafaxine.

SSRI discontinuation syndrome may be avoided by gradual discontinuation of SSRI AD drugs over 6–8 weeks. Some patients may require gradual discontinuation of treatment over several months. In the event that even very gradual withdrawal of treatment leads to discontinuation syndrome switching to treatment with fluoxetine and gradually withdrawing it over several months is usually effective. Liquid formulations of AD drugs permit very gradual withdrawal. A discontinuation syndrome has also been described for TCA and MAOI AD drugs.

Despite a significant proportion of patients experiencing discontinuation syndrome there is no clear evidence that craving, tolerance and addiction occur with SSRI or other newer AD drugs.

Selective serotonin reuptake inhibitors

SSRI AD drugs commonly cause nausea, dyspepsia, crampy abdominal pain and diarrhoea during the initial weeks of treatment and all patients should be warned of this possibility. Tolerance to these adverse effects develops rapidly and they will disappear in most patients after 7–10 days of treatment. In contrast, if headache or excessive nocturnal sweating occurs, it is likely to persist and treatment with an alternative AD drug may be necessary.

SSRI AD drugs may cause mild anorexia and weight loss, although paroxetine may be associated with weight gain.

Sexual dysfunction (diminished libido, erectile and ejaculatory impotence and anorgasmia) is much more common with SSRI AD drugs than with TCA AD drugs and may affect as many as 1 in 3 patients. This is not usually a problem during the acute phase of treatment but is a major cause of treatment discontinuation in the later stages of recovery and during prophylaxis.

The effect of SSRI AD drugs on the fetus has been investigated. Hallberg (2005) reported congenital malformations in 2.9% of infants born to 4291 mothers exposed to SSRI AD drugs during pregnancy versus an expected rate of 3.5% in unexposed infants. Given this and similar studies it is generally accepted that SSRI AD drugs may be prescribed during pregnancy only if the potential benefit outweighs the potential risk to mother and fetus. This is particularly the case given that a recent retrospective study of infants born to 3581 mothers exposed to AD drugs during early pregnancy suggests a doubling of the risk of congenital malformations for paroxetine compared to other AD drugs (FDA 2005). Babies born to women who have taken SSRI AD drugs during the third trimester may experience tremor, restlessness and rigidity in the days immediately following their birth.

Less common adverse effects associated with SSRI AD drugs include:

- Psychomotor arousal (which may be an advantage to some patients).
- Extrapyramidal syndromes including acute dystonia, Parkinsonism and tardive dyskinesia occur rarely with SSRI AD drugs but nonetheless more commonly than with TCA AD drugs. Orofacial dystonia has been reported with paroxetine.
- Hyponatraemia, especially in older patients and possibly due to inappropriate secretion of antidiuretic hormone, has been reported with all AD drugs, especially SSRI AD drugs. The CSM advise that this possibility should be considered in all patients taking an AD drug who become drowsy or confused or who experience seizures.
- Serotonin syndrome, characterised by confusion, fever, myoclonus, chorea, seizures and coma. This also occurs with venlafaxine. It is more likely to occur if SSRI AD drugs or SNRI AD drugs are administered in combination with MAOI AD drugs.
- Seizures may also occur.

In contrast to TCA AD drugs, SSRI AD drugs have no effect on cardiac function and are safe in overdosage, a fact well illustrated by Henry's 1997 report of approximately 14–48 and 1–6 deaths per million prescriptions for TCA AD drugs and SSRI AD drugs (and lofepramine) respectively.

Serotonin and noradrenaline (norepinephrine) reuptake inhibitors

The adverse effects described above for the SSRI drugs may also be experienced by patients taking SNRI drugs. In addition, venlafaxine is contraindicated in patients with heart disease, electrolyte imbalance or hypertension and it may cause alterations in dreaming in some patients.

Reversible monoamine oxidase type A inhibitors

Moclobemide may cause tremor and confusion but is not associated with the specific MAOI adverse effects described below.

Miscellaneous newer antidepressant drugs

Mirtazapine may pose a higher risk for weight gain and blood dyscrasias than other AD drugs.

Tryptophan is thought to be associated with the autoimmune disorder eosinophilia myalgia syndrome although there is evidence that it is not tryptophan itself but rather a contaminant (peak X) that is generated during its manufacture that is responsible (see Table 9.2).

The symptoms of this occasionally fatal syndrome include severe myalgia or arthralgia, fever, dyspnoea, neuropathy, peripheral oedema and skin lesions (sclerosis or papular and urticarial lesions). Eosinophils are elevated to above $1.0 \times 10^9/l$.

Older antidepressant drugs

Tricyclic antidepressant drugs

TCA AD drugs are potent NA α_1, Ach muscarinic M_1 and histamine H_1 neuroreceptor antagonists. Some are also DA D_2 antagonists. These properties alone and in combination, and other as yet poorly understood central mechanisms, are responsible for the adverse effects presented in Table 9.3. It is thought that the general increase in noradrenergic tone associated with TCA AD drugs is responsible for the anxiety, agitation, tremor and increased sweating experienced by some patients. TCA AD drugs also inhibit fast Na^+ channels in the heart and thus have Class I (membrane stabilising) antiarrhythmic properties. These may occasionally cause heart block in healthy individuals but effects are usually of no clinical significance at therapeutic dosages. In overdose, however, TCA AD drugs are highly cardiotoxic because:

- a reservoir of potentially absorbable drug remains available in the proximal small intestine for a prolonged period because their Ach muscarinic M_1 antagonist effects delay gastrointestinal motility
- their Class I antiarrhythmic properties slow ventricular conduction and thus promote ventricular tachyarrhythmias and
- they impair alveolar gas exchange and cause hypoxia, hypercapnia and acidosis and acidosis in turn reduces protein binding and increases available free TCA AD drug.

As is the case with many drugs, TCA AD drugs may cause rashes, hypersensitivity reactions, leucopaenia, agranulocytosis, eosinophilia, thrombocytopaenia and hyponatraemia (especially in older patients and possibly due to inappropriate secretion of antidiuretic hormone). Neuroleptic malignant syndrome occurs rarely (see Chapter 8).

Tricyclic-related antidepressant drugs

The TCA-related AD drugs have adverse effects similar to those of the TCA AD drugs. Mianserin and trazodone are relatively free of cardiovascular adverse effects but are associated with increased risks of white cell dyscrasias and priapism respectively.

Table 9.3: Adverse effects attributable to the antagonism of tricyclic antidepressant drugs at different neuroreceptors

Neuroreceptor antagonism	Adverse effect
Noradrenergic α_1	Dizziness, postural hypotension (may lead to falls and hip fractures in older patients), sexual dysfunction, dry mouth, constipation
Cholinergic muscarinic M_1	Dry mouth, constipation (occasionally, paralytic ileus in older patients), dry eyes, blurred vision, closed angle glaucoma, urinary hesitancy, urinary retention (especially in males with prostatic hypertrophy), sexual dysfunction, mild tachycardia (because of reduced vagal tone), impaired memory and confusion
Histaminergic H_1	Sedation (may be a benefit for some patients but may also impair occupational and driving ability), weight gain (antiserotonergic mechanisms also implicated)
Dopaminergic D_2	Extrapyramidal syndromes, hyperprolactinaemia (especially likely with amoxapine and clomipramine)
Complex central mechanisms	Lowered seizure threshold with increased risk of epileptic seizures, induction of manic episode (more likely in patients with recognised or unrecognised bipolar disorder)

Monoamine oxidase inhibitor drugs

MAOI AD drugs may cause a potentially fatal hypertensive crisis because they inactivate MAO in the gut and prevent the neutralisation of ingested sympathomimetic substances (dietary tyramine and histamine and drugs such as phenylpropanolamine and ephedrine). Patients being treated with MAOI AD drugs must be warned against:

- eating foods including some extracts (meat, soya or yeast), mature cheeses, pickled herring and broad bean pods
- drinking full-bodied red wines and
- taking over-the-counter cough remedies containing phenylpropanolamine and ephedrine.

These dietary restrictions apply both during treatment and for 2 weeks after treatment is discontinued. They do not apply to patients treated with the RIMA, moclobemide.

The general adverse effects associated with MAOI AD drugs include hypotension, insomnia and psychomotor arousal. They may also cause dry mouth, constipation, urinary hesitancy and retention, sexual dysfunction and confusion despite having no anticholinergic properties. They have no effect on cardiac function. They may also induce manic episode, even in patients who do not have bipolar disorder. Phenelzine is a rare cause of peripheral neuropathy.

References and further reading

Altschuler L, Suppes T, Black D et al (2003) Impact of antidepressant discontinuation after acute bipolar depression remission on rates of depressive relapse at 1-year follow-up. American Journal of Psychiatry 160(7):1252–1262.

Cleare (2005) Unipolar depression. In: Core Psychiatry (Eds Wright P, Stern J, Phelan M) (2nd Edition). Elsevier Saunders, Edinburgh, pp. 271–294.

Committee on Safety of Medicines (2005) Safety of selective serotonin reuptake inhibitor antidepressants (CEM/CMO/2004/11) http://medicines.mhra.gov.uk/aboutagency/regframework/csm/csmhome.htm (accessed July 2005).

Coppen A (1967) The biochemistry of affective disorders. British Journal of Psychiatry 113:1237–1264.

Delgado PL, Miller HL, Salomon RM et al (1999) Tryptophan-depletion challenge in depressed patients treated with desipramine or fluoxetine: implications for the role of serotonin in the mechanism of antidepressant action. Biological Psychiatry 46(2):212–220.

FDA 2005 available on line at: www.fda.gov/medwatch/safety/2005/Paxil_dearhcp_letter.pdf [Accessed December 2005]

Fountoulakis KN, Vieta E, Sanchez-Moreno J, Kaprinis SG, Goikolea JM, Kaprinis GS (2005) Treatment guidelines for bipolar disorder: a critical review. Journal of Affective Disorders 86(1):1–10.

Geddes JR, Carney SM, Davies C et al (2003) Relapse prevention with antidepressant drug treatment in depressive disorders: a systematic review. Lancet 361: 653–661.

Hallberg P, Sjoblom V (2005) The use of selective serotonin reuptake inhibitors during pregnancy and breast-feeding: a review and clinical aspects. Journal of Clinical Psychopharmacology 25(1):59–73.

Henry J (1997) Fatal toxicity index. Drug Safety 16: 374–390.

Jamison KR (2000) Suicide and bipolar disorder. Journal of Clinical Psychiatry 61(Suppl 9):47–51.

Judd LL, Akiskal HS, Schettler PJ et al (2002) The long-term natural history of the weekly symptomatic status of bipolar I disorder. Archives of General Psychiatry 59(6):530–537.

Kessler RC, McGonagle KA, Zhao S et al (1994) Lifetime and 12-month prevalence of DSM-III-R psychiatric disorders in the United States. Results from the National Comorbidity Survey. Archives of General Psychiatry 51(1):8–19.

Maes M, Meltzer H (1997) The serotonin hypothesis of major depression. In: Psychopharmacology: Fourth Generation of Progress (Eds Bloom FE, Kupfer DJ). New York, Raven Press, pp. 933–944.

National Institute for Clinical Excellence – Management of depression in primary and secondary care (Dec 2004) available online at http://www.nice.org.uk/pdf/word/CG023NICEguideline.doc (accessed July 2005).

Peet M (1994) Induction of mania with selective serotonin re-uptake inhibitors and tricyclic antidepressants. British Journal of Psychiatry 164(4):549–550.

Wong DT, Bymaster F (2002) Dual serotonin and noradrenaline uptake inhibitor class of antidepressants – potential for greater efficacy or just hype? In: Progress in Drug Research (Ed. Jucker T). Basel, Birkhauser Verlag AG. pp. 169–222.

10

Antimanic and mood stabilising drugs

Introduction

The treatment of bipolar disorder may be divided into three overlapping phases, the treatment of acute mania or manic episode, the treatment of depressive episode (or bipolar depression) and prophylactic treatment intended to prevent recurrence of further manic or depressive episodes.

Acute mania (manic episode)

The antimanic drugs include the antipsychotic (AP) and benzodiazepine (BZD) drugs along with lithium, valproate and carbamazepine (Keck, 2003). The AP and BZD drugs are discussed in Chapters 8 and 11 respectively. An account of lithium is provided below while valproate and carbamazepine are discussed in Chapter 12.

The pharmacological treatment of acute mania is largely determined by the severity of an individual patient's symptoms.

Moderate or severe acute mania

Patients with moderate or severe acute mania frequently require hospitalisation and this often has to be effected under mental health legislation. Treatment is essential in order to:

- reduce the patient's agitation and distress
- rapidly control their behaviour and thus reduce risk to the patient and others

- initiate the treatment of psychotic symptoms and
- prevent further episodes of acute mania in the longer term.

AP drugs significantly reduce manic symptoms in 1–2 days while lithium takes 1–2 weeks to have the same effect. Valproate and carbamazepine are effective in an intermediate timeframe of perhaps 1 week. AP drugs are therefore generally regarded as the most appropriate initial treatment for acute mania.

Guidance on the treatment of bipolar disorder will not be available from the National Institute for Clinical Excellence (NICE) until late 2006 although it should be noted that a NICE technology appraisal recommends the use of olanzapine and valproate semisodium in acute mania (2003). In the meantime it seems appropriate to extrapolate from NICE guidance on the treatment of schizophrenia and to recommend that the vast majority of patients with moderate or severe acute mania should be treated with atypical AP drugs (2002). These may be administered as monotherapy or, in the case of more agitated patients, in combination with BZD drugs (Goodwin and Young, 2003).

Parenteral administration of medication may be required, either because rapid control of the patient's behaviour must be accomplished in order to reduce risk or, more frequently, because patients do not appreciate that they are ill and in need of treatment and consequently refuse oral therapy. Again it seems appropriate to extrapolate from NICE guidance on the treatment of schizophrenia if parenteral medication is to be administered to a patient with acute mania (2002). Thus it is recommended that:

- intramuscular administration of medication is preferred to intravenous administration on grounds of patient safety
- the intramuscular drugs recommended for use are haloperidol, lorazepam and olanzapine
- a single drug is preferred to a combination of drugs whenever possible and
- if haloperidol (or another typical antipsychotic drug) is administered intramuscularly, an antimuscarinic drug should also be administered in order to reduce the risk of acute dystonia and other EPS side-effects.

Mild acute mania

Patients with mild or less severe acute mania may be treated with either lithium or carbamazepine administered as monotherapy, or with modest doses of atypical AP drugs. Patients who do not respond adequately to atypical AP drugs or to lithium may respond to sodium valproate or to carbamazepine.

Treatment-resistant acute mania

Approximately half of all patients with acute mania will not respond adequately to the treatments described above. Such patients may respond to combination therapy consisting of an atypical AP drug and either lithium or carbamazepine. Clozapine has also been used successfully to treat patients with acute mania which has proved resistant to AP drugs alone and in combination with lithium or carbamazepine. As noted in Chapter 17, a small proportion of patients with acute mania require treatment with electroconvulsive therapy (ECT) and this use of ECT is endorsed by NICE (2003).

Even while a patient with acute mania is being treated consideration must be given to long-term prophylactic treatment with a mood stabilising drug so that in as far as it is possible recurrences of either manic or depressive episodes are prevented.

Bipolar depressive episode (bipolar depression)

The treatment of bipolar depressive episode or bipolar depression is described in Chapter 9.

Prophylactic treatment in bipolar disorder

The importance of prophylactic treatment with mood stabilising drugs in bipolar disorder cannot be doubted. Prospective naturalistic investigations, in which patients receive standard treatment with which they may or may not comply, have reported relapse rates of over 40% after 1 year and almost 90% after 5 years. Relapse rates in patients treated with placebo (in the context of double-blind clinical trials) are in excess of 80% after 1 year (Tohen et al, 2005).

Mood stabilising drugs

There is no satisfactory definition of a mood stabilising drug. Ideally, a mood stabilising drug should effectively treat and effectively prevent both acute mania and bipolar depression. None of the drugs currently regarded as mood stabilising drugs fulfil these criteria.

The mood stabilising drugs that are currently available include lithium salts, the antiepileptic drugs valproate, carbamazepine and lamotrigine (see Chapter 12) and the atypical AP olanzapine (see Chapter 8) (Goodwin and Young, 2003). The regulatory status of these drugs in the UK is currently as follows:

- Lithium salts are approved for 'the treatment and prophylaxis of mania, manic-depressive illness and recurrent depression'.
- Valproate semisodium is approved for 'the acute treatment of a manic episode associated with bipolar disorder' while sodium valproate is not currently approved for administration to patients with bipolar disorder.
- Carbamazepine is approved for 'the prophylaxis of manic-depressive psychosis in patients unresponsive to lithium therapy'.
- Lamotrigine is not currently approved for administration to patients with bipolar disorder.
- Olanzapine is approved for 'the treatment of moderate to severe manic episode' and 'the prevention of recurrence in patients with bipolar disorder'.

Thus only lithium and olanzapine are approved in the UK as first-line prophylactic treatments in bipolar disorder while carbamazepine is approved as a second-line prophylactic treatment in patients who do not respond to lithium.

General efficacy of mood stabilising drugs

Prophylactic mood stabilising drugs are recommended for patients who have experienced either:

- a single manic episode that caused significant personal (for example attempted suicide, criminal convictions, loss of driving licence, sexually transmitted disease, significant debt), domestic (for example divorce, marital disharmony) or occupational (for example inability to continue education or career, medical retirement, prolonged absence from work) impact
- two manic episodes or
- an episode of mania and an episode of depression.

Some patients with recurrent depressive illness also benefit from mood stabilising drugs as do some patients with psychotic disorders such as schizophrenia, especially when a significant affective component is present. Lithium is also employed in the treatment of aggression and self-mutilating behaviour.

Lithium salts have been the mainstay of prophylactic monotherapy in bipolar disorder for almost four decades. However, almost one in three patients relapse while taking lithium. Such patients have historically been treated with valproate or carbamazepine, either alone or in combination with lithium salts, but olanzapine and lamotrigine are increasingly prescribed in this situation.

Historically, it has been usual practice to gradually withdraw the AP drugs prescribed to treat patients with acute mania once prophylactic treatment with a mood stabilising drug has been established and their symptoms have resolved. This was largely because the typical AP drugs that were utilised carry a significant risk for tardive dyskinesia. Nonetheless, the typical AP drugs – including depot formulations – represent the third line of prophylactic treatment in patients with bipolar disorder.

The atypical AP drugs carry a low risk for tardive dyskinesia and olanzapine, quetiapine and risperidone have recently been approved for the treatment of acute mania. Olanzapine is also approved for the prevention of recurrence in patients with bipolar disorder (see above). The possibility of treating a patient during a manic episode with an atypical AP drug that may be continued for long-term prophylaxis seems attractive, especially when such drugs do not require blood testing. However, it remains to be seen if the atypical AP drugs become established as first-line mood stabilising drugs.

General safety of mood stabilising drugs

When selecting a mood stabilising drug it should be borne in mind that treatment will continue indefinitely and may be lifelong. The adverse effects of such drugs and their impact on patients' lives, and thus on compliance with treatment, must therefore be carefully considered and fully discussed with every patient.

Psychopharmacology and our understanding of bipolar disorder

While an understanding of the mechanism of action of AP and AD drugs has greatly increased our understanding of schizophrenia and depression, the contribution of psychopharmacology to our understanding of bipolar disorder has been more modest.

AP drugs effectively treat acute mania and it is assumed by extrapolation from schizophrenia that the mechanism of action is dopamine (DA) D_2 neuroreceptor antagonism. But lithium and antiepileptic drugs which have no effect at the DA D_2 neuroreceptor are also effective treatments for acute mania. Similarly, AD drugs effectively treat bipolar depression and it is assumed by extrapolation from major depressive disorder that the mechanism of action in bipolar depression is enhanced serotonergic and/or noradrenergic neurotransmission. But lithium, antiepileptic drugs and olanzapine, which have little effect on serotonergic and/or noradrenergic neurotransmission, prevent depressive relapse in bipolar depression but not in major depressive disorder.

It is intriguing that drugs with such different mechanisms of action as AP drugs (DA D_2 neuroreceptor antagonism), antiepileptic drugs (valproate causes upregulation of gamma-amino butyric acid ($GABA_B$) receptors, carbamazepine blocks N-methyl, D-aspartate (NMDA) receptors and lamotrigine blocks fast sodium channels – see Chapter 12) and lithium (which causes neither DA D_2 neuroreceptor antagonism, upregulation of $GABA_B$ receptors, blockade of NMDA receptors nor blockade of fast sodium channels) are all effective in preventing relapse in bipolar disorder.

The modest contribution of psychopharmacology to our understanding of bipolar disorder is compounded by our lack of understanding of the mechanism of action of lithium (see below).

Lithium

The discovery of the efficacy of lithium salts in the treatment of acute mania and of their subsequent clinical development as mood stabilising drugs has been described in Chapter 2.

Pharmacokinetics

Lithium is an alkali metal that may be administered as either its lithium carbonate or its lithium citrate salt. The active component of both is the lithium cation (Li^+).

Lithium:

- is rapidly and completely absorbed at the proximal small intestine and, to a lesser extent, the stomach

- reaches C_{MAX} in 1–2 hours and has a $T_{1/2}$ of approximately 24 hours (these parameters would normally militate against once daily dosing because the dose required to maintain an effective blood level throughout the day would result in toxicity at C_{MAX}. However, currently available tablets are coated so as to delay absorption and produce a non-toxic C_{MAX} approximately 4 hours after administration and effective blood levels throughout the day. This also means that the available preparations differ significantly in bioavailability)

- is not metabolised (it is an element) and is eliminated unchanged via the kidney

- is minimally bound to plasma proteins and

- has a narrow therapeutic window, being largely ineffective at serum levels below 0.4 mmol/l and toxic at levels above 1.5 mmol/l (see below).

Pharmacodynamics

The mechanism of action of lithium is unknown. It has been suggested that it may stabilise neuronal membranes by substituting for other cations (it is known that it alters sodium transport in neurones), or modify neuronal second messenger systems by inhibiting inositol monophosphatase, the enzyme responsible for the metabolism of phosphatidylinositol. An effect of lithium on gene expression via modulation of protein kinase C has also been proposed.

Efficacy

Lithium is approved in the UK for the 'treatment and prophylaxis of mania, manic-depressive illness and recurrent depression'. It is a second-line (after continuation of treatment with a newer type of AD drug) or adjuvant treatment for the prevention of new depressive episodes in major depressive disorder. Lithium may also be used to control aggressive or self-mutilating behaviour.

The daily dosage should be increased gradually until serum lithium measured 12 hours after administration is maintained in the range 0.4–1.0 mmol/l. It was previously recommended to maintain serum lithium measured 12 hours after administration in the range 0.6–1.2 mmol/l but this is now regarded as excessive for most patients. A range of 0.4–0.7 mmol/l is appropriate for elderly patients.

It is usual to measure serum lithium weekly while the dose is being titrated to the therapeutic range and every 3 months thereafter. The daily dosage may be divided during the initial titration phase but once daily administration is usual when an individual patient's daily dose has been established. Patients taking lithium require baseline and regular laboratory investigations in addition to serum lithium assays (see below).

The most recently reported investigation of lithium in the prophylaxis of bipolar disorder is that of Tohen et al (2005) who compared it with olanzapine in a randomised, double-blind trial in 431 patients that extended over one year. Relapse occurred in 38.8% of the lithium-treated and 30.0% of the olanzapine-treated patients. Manic relapse occurred in 23.4% of the lithium-treated and 13.8% of the olanzapine-treated patients, while depressive relapse occurred in 10.7% of the lithium-treated and 15.7% of the olanzapine-treated patients. This study confirms the efficacy of both lithium and olanzapine as prophylactic treatments in bipolar disorder.

Approximately 50% of patients in whom treatment with lithium is abruptly discontinued will develop mania, often referred to as rebound mania, within 1–2 weeks (Verdoux and Bourgeois, 1993). Rebound mania may be avoided by gradual discontinuation of lithium over 6–8 weeks if treatment must cease.

Safety

Even when their serum lithium levels are maintained within the therapeutic range the majority of patients taking lithium experience adverse effects. These adverse effects – some of which worsen as serum lithium levels increase and thus may warn of lithium toxicity (see below) – may be classified by the body systems affected by them as follows.

Central nervous system

Dysphoria, emotional and cognitive dulling, especially memory impairment (these are complained of by many patients and are a frequent cause of non-adherence to treatment) and tremor (a high-frequency, low-amplitude tremor which embarrasses many patients, becomes more evident as serum lithium increases and may predict toxicity. A moderately objective measure of the presence and severity of tremor may be obtained by observing changes in patients' signatures – written in their medical records at each clinic appointment – over time).

Endocrine and reproductive systems

Asymptomatic goitre, hypothyroidism (thyroid function should be evaluated every 6–12 months) and teratogenicity. There is an increased risk of cardiac malformations, especially Ebstein's anomaly, if lithium is taken in the months before conception and/or during the first trimester. There is some evidence that lithium is not a major teratogen (Jacobson et al, 1992) but women taking lithium should plan their pregnancies and should discontinue it before conception and as a minimum during the first trimester. Lithium is secreted in breast milk and may cause neonatal hypothyroidism in breastfed babies.

Genitourinary system

Polyuria, increased urinary output and nephrogenic diabetes insipidus (lithium inhibits the action of antidiuretic hormone at the renal tubule). Oedema may also occur and may increase the risk of lithium toxicity if treated with diuretics (see below).

Gastrointestinal system

Increased or decreased salivation, metallic taste (caused by secretion of lithium in saliva), polydipsia (in response to polyuria), nausea, vomiting, epigastric discomfort, mild diarrhoea and weight gain.

Skin

Rash, exacerbation of existing or development of *de novo* psoriasis and hair loss.

Cardiovascular system

Clinically insignificant flattening or inverting of T waves on ECG and, rarely, symptomatic conduction defects.

Lithium toxicity

Lithium toxicity is evident in some patients with serum lithium levels of 1.5 mmol/l and in almost all with levels greater than 2.0 mmol/l. It usually develops over 1–2 days and may be precipitated by dehydration, impaired renal function, concomitant infection, treatment with diuretics or deliberate overdose. Elderly patients are particularly liable to lithium toxicity.

The adverse effects that may be present in the non-toxic state worsen at the onset of lithium toxicity and patients initially experience severe vomiting and diarrhoea, marked thirst, polydipsia and polyuria. They also develop a coarse tremor. With increasing toxicity, the clinical picture progresses through hypertonicity, choreoathetoid movements, ataxia and dysarthria to delirium, seizures, renal failure and impaired consciousness. Untreated, cardiovascular collapse, coma and death soon follow.

Toxicity may be prevented by advising patients of the importance of hydration and by temporarily discontinuing lithium and encouraging hydration at the first signs of toxicity. There is no specific antidote for lithium toxicity and established toxicity should be treated by discontinuing lithium, forcing diuresis and maintaining electrolyte balance. Some patients will require peritoneal dialysis or haemodialysis, control of seizures and other supportive measures.

References and further reading

Goodwin GM, Young AH (2003) The British Association for Psychopharmacology guidelines for treatment of bipolar disorder: a summary. Journal of Psychopharmacology 17(4)(Suppl):3–6.

Jacobson SJ, Jones K, Johnson K, et al (1992) Prospective multicentre study of pregnancy outcome after lithium exposure during first trimester. Lancet 339(8792):530–533.

Keck PE (2003) The management of acute mania. British Medical Journal 327:1002–1003.

National Institute for Clinical Excellence (2002) Schizophrenia: Core Interventions in the Treatment and Management of Schizophrenia in Primary and Secondary Care. Available at: www.nice.org.uk (accessed July 2005).

National Institute for Clinical Excellence (2003) Olanzapine and valproate semisodium in the treatment of acute mania associated with bipolar I disorder. Available at: www.nice.org.uk (accessed July 2005).

National Institute for Clinical Excellence (2003) Guidance on the use of electroconvulsive therapy. Available at: www.nice.org.uk (accessed July 2005).

Tohen M, Greil W, Calabrese JR, et al (2005) Olanzapine versus lithium in the maintenance treatment of bipolar disorder: a 12-month, randomized, double-blind, controlled clinical trial. American Journal of Psychiatry 162(7):1281–1290.

Verdoux H, Bourgeois M (1993) Short-term sequelae of lithium discontinuation. Encephale 19(6):645–650.

11

Anxiolytic and hypnotic drugs

Introduction

Humans have always sought relief from both appropriate and inappropriate fear. This search led to the discovery of drugs such as cannabis and opium in the very distant past, to the synthesis of alcohol in the distant past and to the invention of barbiturates and benzodiazepine (BZD) drugs in the last century. More recently it has led to the development of non-BZD drugs and to the use of drugs with primarily antidepressant (AD) properties in the treatment of anxiety disorders.

The BZD and non-BZD anxiolytic and hypnotic drugs will now be discussed and this will be followed by a description of the use of AD drugs in the treatment of anxiety disorders.

Benzodiazepine drugs

The barbiturates and meprobamate (which is still available – see below) were the most widely prescribed drugs of the 1940s and 1950s respectively. However, their propensity to cause dependence stimulated a search for drugs with similar 'tranquillising' properties but without this risk. The first BZD compound was discovered in 1957, chlordiazepoxide was provided for clinical use in 1960 and diazepam followed in 1962 (see Chapter 2).

The BZD drugs were to prove very effective as tranquillisers and their use expanded rapidly through the 1960s and 1970s. By then, it was realised that the BZD drugs were as likely to cause dependence as their predecessors and the last two decades have seen attempts to curb widespread prescribing. Nonetheless, the BZD drugs remain the most widely prescribed treatments for anxiety and insomnia.

The BZD drugs available in the UK include alprazolam, chlordiazepoxide, clobazam, clonazepam, clorazepate, diazepam, flurazepam, loprazolam, lorazepam, lormetazepam, midazolam, nitrazepam, oxazepam and temazepam. Many more are available in other countries.

BZD drugs are structurally similar and have in common a benzene ring attached to a diazepine ring (hence benzodiazepine) which in turn is attached to a phenyl ring. In general, individual BZD drugs differ from each other structurally in the side chains that are attached to their diazepine rings.

Pharmacokinetics

It is convenient to consider the pharmacokinetics of BZD drugs under the headings of absorption, metabolism and plasma protein binding and of duration of pharmacological action.

Absorption, metabolism and plasma protein binding

Individual BZD drugs differ in the rate at which they are absorbed from the gastrointestinal tract. Diazepam and flurazepam are rapidly absorbed, for example, and reach C_{MAX} in approximately 1 hour. Temazepam, in contrast, is absorbed slowly and does not reach C_{MAX} for at least 3 hours. Liquid formulations of BZD drugs are absorbed rapidly if administered rectally, C_{MAX} being reached in 15–30 minutes. This route of administration is of practical use in the control of epileptic seizures in children.

Absorption of BZD drugs following intramuscular (IM) injection is erratic for reasons that are not well understood and it is best not to administer BZD drugs by this route. However, while it is generally true that the IM route has no therapeutic advantage over the oral route, it may be necessary to administer BZD drugs IM if it is not possible to do so by the oral or intravenous (IV) routes.

BZD drugs are metabolised in the liver, often with the production of active metabolites (see below), by:

- simple conjugation with glucuronic acid to produce water-soluble glucuronides that are excreted by the kidney or by
- complex pathways with several steps, for example demethylation or dealkylation followed by glucuronidation.

Plasma protein binding of BZD drugs is generally in excess of 90%. The exception to this rule is alprazolam for which plasma protein binding is 75%.

Individual BZD drugs differ significantly in their lipid solubility. This is lowest for lorazepam and temazepam, twice as great for diazepam and three times as great for midazolam. Midazolam therefore crosses the blood–brain barrier very rapidly and is generally employed to induce anaesthesia.

Duration of pharmacological action

The half lives ($T_{1/2}$) of individual BZD drugs differ dramatically and this, and the fact that many have active metabolites with long $T_{1/2}$ of their own, complicates their clinical use. Flurazepam, for example, has a $T_{1/2}$ of 1–2 hours but its active metabolite, desalkylflurazepam, has a $T_{1/2}$ of 75 hours. Flurazepam therefore has a longer effective $T_{1/2}$ than the $T_{1/2}$ of the parent compound would suggest. Similarly chlordiazepoxide and diazepam with $T_{1/2}$ of 15 and 20–100 hours respectively both have desmethyldiazepam with a $T_{1/2}$ of 80 hours as an active metabolite.

It is useful to classify BZD drugs into those with very short, short, medium and long durations of action as presented in Table 11.1 by consideration of the following:

- the $T_{1/2}$ of the parent drug
- the $T_{1/2}$ of any active metabolite(s) and
- in the case of oxazepam, lorazepam and temazepam, the absence of active metabolites.

In general, the BZD drugs listed in Table 11.1 as having very short and short durations of action are useful hypnotics that cause little daytime sedation. They do, however, carry a significant risk of causing physical and psychological dependence.

Table 11.1: Benzodiazepine drugs with very short, short, medium and long durations of action and their usual clinical applications

Hypnotics		Anxiolytics	
Very short	**Short**	**Medium**	**Long**
Loprazolam	Flurazepam[1]	Alprazolam	Clorazepate
Lormetazepam	Nitrazepam	Lorazepam	Chlordiazepoxide
Temazepam		Midazolam[2]	Clobazam
		Oxazepam	Clonazepam
			Diazepam

Notes:
[1]See commentary on the $T_{1/2}$ of flurazepam above.
[2]Midazolam is employed to induce anaesthesia and is not widely used in psychiatric practice.

In contrast, the BZD drugs listed in Table 11.1 as having medium and long durations of action are useful anxiolytic drugs. And while they have a tendency to cause daytime sedation which may be a problem for drivers and those who operate machinery, they have a reduced propensity for inducing physical and psychological dependence.

Pharmacodynamics

Gamma-amino butyric acid (GABA) is the main inhibitory neuro-transmitter in the brain and BZD drugs are potent postsynaptic $GABA_A$ receptor agonists. It is thought that $GABA_A$ receptors possess two binding sites, one for GABA, the natural ligand, on the β protein subunit and the other for BZD drugs, synthetic ligands, on the α protein subunit (Fig. 11.1). Physiologically, GABA binds to the β subunit of the $GABA_A$ receptor. This causes the ion channel to open and allows the influx of chloride ions (Cl^-) into the neurone. The excess negative charge generated by the Cl^- ions causes hyperpolarisation of the neurone and prevents it from reaching action potential.

BZD drugs bind to the α subunit of the $GABA_A$ receptor. This has no direct effect on the ion channel but it alters the β subunit and facilitates its ability to bind GABA. This in turn causes the ion channel to open. BZD drugs have no effect on $GABA_A$ receptors in the absence of GABA. Thus binding of a BZD drug such as diazepam to the $GABA_A$ receptor enhances the effect of GABA and causes a greater influx of Cl^- than is possible through binding of GABA alone. This synergy between natural and synthetic ligands is an example of allosteric modulation (see Chapter 3).

$GABA_A$ receptors are present throughout the brain but it is believed that BZD drugs exert their anxiolytic and anticonvulsant effects by facilitating GABA-induced neuronal inhibition at specific neuro-anatomical sites. The nature of this specificity is not understood. However, it is known that $GABA_A$ receptors with many different amino acid sequences exist and it is believed that at least a few of these differ both in their neuroanatomical distribution and in their function (see Chapter 3). Thus:

- the highest concentration of $GABA_A$ BZD-1 (also referred to as the $GABA_A$ α_1 or the omega-1) receptors is in the cerebellum. These are believed to mediate the anxiolytic and hypnotic effects of BZD drugs while

- the highest concentration of $GABA_A$ BZD-2 (also referred to as the $GABA_A$ α_2 or the omega-2) receptors is in the striatum and these are believed to mediate the muscle-relaxant effects of BZD drugs.

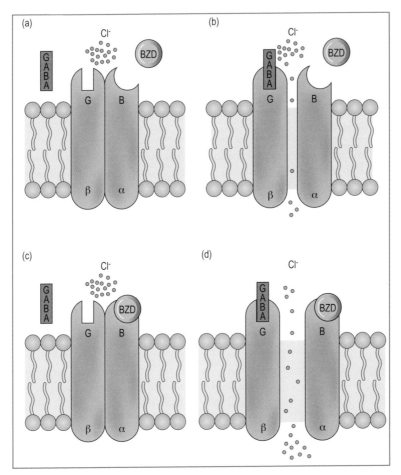

Fig. 11.1 Mechanism of action of benzodiazepine drugs at the GABA$_A$ receptor.
(**a**) GABA$_A$ receptors possess two binding sites, one for GABA, the natural ligand, on
the β protein subunit (G) and the other for BZD drugs, synthetic ligands, on the
α protein subunit (B). (**b**) When GABA binds to the β subunit of the GABA$_A$ receptor
the ion channel opens and chloride ions (Cl⁻) enter the neurone. This generates an
excess negative charge which hyperpolarises the neurone and prevents it from
reaching action potential. (**c**) When BZD drugs bind to the α subunit of the GABA$_A$
receptor they have no direct effect on the function of the ion channel. (**d**) However,
BZD drugs binding to the α subunit of the GABA$_A$ receptor alter the β subunit and
facilitate its ability to bind GABA. This causes the ion channel to open to a greater
extent than occurs through binding of GABA alone. This in turn permits a greater
influx of Cl⁻ into the neurone than is possible through binding of GABA alone
(allosteric modulation).

BZD drugs bind indiscriminately to both GABA$_A$ BZD-1 and GABA$_A$ BZD-2 receptors while non-BZD anxiolytic and hypnotic drugs such as zaleplon, zolpidem and zopiclone bind preferentially to the GABA$_A$ BZD-1 receptor (see below). It is also thought that an as yet unidentified endogenous ligand or 'endozepine' may exist for the α subunit of the GABA$_A$ receptor.

Efficacy

BZD drugs are indicated at the lowest effective dose and for the shortest possible time for the treatment of severe anxiety disorders and severe insomnia. They should not be prescribed for mild anxiety or mild insomnia.

BZD drugs are also useful in psychiatric emergencies and in epilepsy (see Chapter 12) and have many uses as sedatives in general medicine and in dentistry.

Anxiety disorders

BZD drugs with long durations of action may be used to prevent severe anxiety occurring in response to a discrete stimulus. Severe anxiety induced by fear of air travel, for example, may be prevented by 2–5 mg of diazepam or 10–15 mg chlordiazepoxide administered as a single dose a few hours before the flight. This represents a reasonable use of BZD drugs given that air travel is a relatively infrequent undertaking for most people. Dependence is therefore unlikely to develop and the use of a BZD may permit a business trip or holiday.

Chronic anxiety disorders such as panic disorder and generalised anxiety disorder also respond to BZD drugs with long durations of action. Short-term treatment (2–4 weeks) of such disorders is appropriate while awaiting a safer long-term treatment such as a selective serotonin reuptake inhibitor (SSRI) or cognitive therapy or both to take effect. Long-term treatment with BZD drugs should be guarded against because it carries with it the risk of dependence and tolerance with patients requiring ever increasing doses of drug in order to obtain the same clinical benefit.

The use of BZD drugs to alleviate distress in bereaved individuals is a widespread practice. However, this is a use that is probably best avoided except in cases of extreme distress because medications are likely to impair the psychological adjustments that are part of the normal grieving process.

Insomnia

Very short-acting BZD drugs may be useful in the short-term (1–3 weeks) treatment of insomnia when initial insomnia is present. Patients in whom insomnia is caused by depression, for example, may benefit from such treatment while awaiting the onset of action of AD drugs. In a similar manner, patients with insomnia for which there is no apparent cause may benefit while awaiting the onset of action of behavioural treatments and educational programmes. Very short-acting BZD drugs may cause withdrawal symptoms but generally do not cause 'hangover' the next day.

Short-acting BZD drugs have a longer duration of action than very short-acting BZD drugs and may be useful in the short-term (1–3 weeks or less) treatment of insomnia when interrupted sleep occurs. They are less likely to cause withdrawal symptoms than very short-acting BZD drugs but may cause 'hangover' the next day.

Equivalent doses

It is often helpful to know the equivalent doses of the different BZD drugs, for example when converting the daily dose of a BZD that a patient is dependent upon to the equivalent daily dose of diazepam in order to facilitate gradual withdrawal. The British National Formulary (2005) gives approximate equivalent doses for diazepam 5 mg as chlordiazepoxide 15 mg, loprazolam 0.5–1.0 mg, lorazepam 0.5 mg, lormetazepam 0.5–1.0 mg, nitrazepam 5 mg, oxazepam 15 mg and temazepam 10 mg.

Safety

BZD drugs are extraordinarily safe. They are effectively free of the adverse effects that may be regarded as common to all drugs (headache, gastrointestinal disturbance), appear to have no cardiac or autonomic effects and even in massive overdose are generally only fatal if taken in combination with other drugs with synergistic effects or with alcohol.

The adverse effects commonly associated with BZD drugs include drowsiness, sedation, dizziness and ataxia. These are significant problems in older patients in whom it may lead to falls and fractures with resultant morbidity and mortality. These adverse effects gradually resolve with continued treatment.

More troublesome is the fact that psychomotor performance is impaired and reaction time increased – adverse effects that drivers and patients who operate machinery must be warned about. Patients must also be warned that these adverse effects are potentiated by alcohol which acts synergistically with BZD drugs and that they may persist for some time as a 'hangover' if BZD drugs with a long duration of action are prescribed.

High doses of BZD drugs administered to BZD naïve patients and/or BZD drugs administered by IV injection may cause respiratory and central nervous system depression. This may be reversed by flumazenil, an imidazobenzodiazepine that is a competitive inhibitor at the α protein subunit of the GABA$_A$ receptor and thus a potent BZD antagonist. It rapidly reverses respiratory and central nervous system depression caused by BZD drugs but caution is required because these may reappear as the effect of flumazenil diminishes.

Paradoxical disinhibition

Patients treated with BZD drugs may appear 'drunk' and this can progress to verbal and physical hostility, especially in the presence of environmental stimuli such as noise or confinement. It is thought that this syndrome occurs because while the dose of BZD prescribed is sufficient to disinhibit and cause 'drunkenness' it is not sufficient to cause tranquillisation. An increase or reduction in the dose will usually resolve the problem.

Tolerance and dependence

It was recognised soon after BZD drugs became available that tolerance (the need for increasingly higher doses to achieve the same clinical effect) to their sedative effects occurs within days or weeks. It was also observed that delirium and seizures may occur if high doses of BZD drugs are abruptly withdrawn. These findings led to attempts to reduce the use of BZD drugs and the number of prescriptions issued has declined in the last decade. Despite this, 12.7 million prescriptions were written for BZD drugs in England in 2002 and more than half of these were prescribed for patients over the age of 65 years.

Dependence seems to occur more readily with BZD drugs which have very short or short durations of action, particularly if their use is prolonged. The treatment of BZD dependence relies upon:

- prevention – local or national prescribing guidelines or those of the Committee on Safety of Medicines (Box 11.1) should be adhered to and
- gradual withdrawal – the daily dose of the BZD the patient is dependent upon should be converted to the equivalent daily dose of diazepam and this dosage gradually reduce over many months. An appropriate rate of diazepam dosage reduction is 1 mg per week or 5 mg per month. A dose should be maintained at any given level if withdrawal syndrome (see below) occurs and only reduced further when it resolves.

Benzodiazepine withdrawal syndrome

The BZD withdrawal syndrome was first described in 1981 (Petursson and Lader). It consists of anxiety, insomnia, weight loss, drowsiness, headache, sweating, myalgia, arthralgia, derealisation, depersonalisation, visual illusions, hyperacusis, tinnitus and paraesthesia. Seizures and a toxic psychosis occur in more severely affected patients. This may

1. Benzodiazepines are indicated for the short-term relief (2–4 weeks only) of anxiety that is severe, disabling or subjecting the individual to unacceptable distress, occurring alone or in association with insomnia or short-term psychosomatic, organic or psychotic illness.
2. The use of benzodiazepines to treat short-term 'mild' anxiety is inappropriate and unsuitable.
3. Benzodiazepines should be used to treat insomnia only when it is severe, disabling, or subjecting the individual to extreme distress.

occur within hours or days in patients abruptly withdrawn from BZD drugs with very short or short durations of action and within days or weeks in patients abruptly withdrawn from BZD drugs with medium or long durations of action. It generally resolves within 2–4 weeks of discontinuing BZD drugs but it may persist for months in some patients.

It should be noted that the symptoms of the BZD withdrawal syndrome are similar to those for which BZD drugs are often prescribed. This may led to further inappropriate prescribing of BZD drugs.

BZD tolerance and dependence, and BZD withdrawal syndrome, may be caused by downregulation in the numbers or sensitivity of $GABA_A$ receptors induced by long-term use of a BZD drug (see Chapter 3). This state would greatly impair GABA-ergic neurotransmission when the BZD drug is withdrawn producing, presumably, the symptoms of the withdrawal syndrome.

Non-benzodiazepine anxiolytic and hypnotic drugs

A number of non-BZD $GABA_A$ receptor agonists have become available in the last decade. These are structurally dissimilar to BZD drugs and include buspirone, zaleplon, zolpidem and zopiclone (the so-called Z-drugs).

The dependence and abuse potential of buspirone is low. Initial hopes that tolerance and a withdrawal syndrome would not occur with zaleplon, zolpidem and zopiclone, and that dependence would not develop, are declining with increasing use of these drugs. The prescribing guidelines applicable to BZD drugs should therefore be followed when they are prescribed. The National Institute for Clinical Excellence (2004) has advised that because of the lack of compelling evidence to distinguish between zaleplon, zolpidem, zopiclone or the shorter-acting benzodiazepine hypnotics, the drug with the lowest purchase cost should be prescribed for the short-term management of insomnia.

Buspirone

Buspirone is an azaspirodecanedione that is approved in the UK for the short-term management of anxiety disorders and the relief of symptoms of anxiety with or without accompanying depression. It is rapidly absorbed, reaching T_{MAX} after approximately 1 hour. It undergoes hepatic metabolism including significant first pass metabolism. Its $T_{1/2}$ is 6 hours.

The mechanism of action of buspirone is not fully understood. It has no affinity for the $GABA_A$ BZD-1 receptor and subsequently does not alleviate the symptoms of BZD withdrawal and has no sedative, antiepileptic or muscle relaxant activity. It is known that it promotes noradrenergic and dopaminergic activity and inhibits serotonergic and cholinergic activity.

Buspirone should be initiated at a dose of 10 to 15 mg daily (administered in 2 or 3 divided doses). The dose may be increased by 5 mg daily every few days to a usual dose of 15 to 30 mg daily and a maximum of 45 mg daily.

Buspirone is contraindicated in epilepsy. It does not cause the cognitive impairment that has been demonstrated with BZD drugs. The commonest adverse effects associated with buspirone are dizziness, headache, nervousness, excitement and nausea. Less frequently, tachycardia, palpitations, chest pain, confusion and seizures occur.

Zaleplon

Zaleplon is a pyrazolopyrimidine that is rapidly and well absorbed, reaching T_{MAX} after 1 hour. It undergoes hepatic metabolism without production of active metabolites. Its $T_{1/2}$ is 1 hour. Zaleplon has high selectivity and low affinity for the $GABA_A$ BZD-1 receptor (80 nM). Its effects are reversed by flumazenil.

Zaleplon in a dose of 10 mg is effective in the treatment of initial insomnia but its short $T_{1/2}$ makes it ineffective in the treatment of interrupted sleep or early morning awakening. Its safety profile is similar to that of BZD drugs.

Zolpidem

Zolpidem is an imidazopyridine that is rapidly and well absorbed, reaching T_{MAX} after 0.5 hours. It undergoes hepatic metabolism without production of active metabolites. Its $T_{1/2}$ is 2.5 hours. Zolpidem has high selectivity for the $GABA_A$ BZD-1 receptor (15 nM). Its effects are reversed by flumazenil.

Zolpidem in a dose of 10 mg is effective in the treatment of initial insomnia and interrupted sleep but its short $T_{1/2}$ make it less effective in the treatment of early morning awakening. Its safety profile is similar to that of BZD drugs.

Zopiclone

Zopiclone is a cyclopyrrolone that is rapidly and well absorbed, reaching T_{MAX} after 0.5 hours. It undergoes hepatic metabolism with production of one slightly active metabolite. Its $T_{1/2}$ is 5 hours. Zopiclone has high selectivity for the $GABA_A$ BZD-1 receptor (50 nM). Its effects are reversed by flumazenil.

Zopiclone's short T_{MAX} and comparatively long $T_{1/2}$ mean it is effective in the treatment of initial insomnia and interrupted sleep, and reasonably effective for early morning wakening, in a dose of 7.5 mg. Its safety profile is similar to that of BZD drugs.

Zaleplon, zolpidem and zopiclone are approved in the UK for the short-term treatment of insomnia. They have very short (zaleplon) or short (zolpidem and zopiclone) durations of action and they are now widely prescribed. Their efficacy and safety is similar to that of BZD drugs. Initial hopes that tolerance and a withdrawal syndrome would not occur and that dependence would not develop are declining as use increases. The prescribing guidelines applicable to BZD drugs should therefore be followed when they are prescribed.

Newer non-benzodiazepine hypnotic drugs

Eszopiclone, the S enantiomer of zopiclone, is approved for the treatment of insomnia for up to 6 months in the US. Its T_{MAX} is 1 hour while its $T_{1/2}$ is 6 hours. It is not currently available in the UK.

Ramelteon has recently been approved for the treatment of insomnia for up to 6 months in the US. Its mechanism of action differs from that of both BZD and non-BZD drugs. It is thought that natural evening sleepiness is triggered by increasing melatonin release from the pineal gland which occurs in response to the effect of diminishing light mediated via the retina and suprachiasmatic nucleus. Ramelteon is an agonist at the G-protein coupled melatonin MT_1 and MT_2 receptors in the suprachiasmatic nucleus where its action is thought to induce sleep by acting as a melatonin analogue.

Other hypnotic and sedative drugs

Chloral hydrate and triclofos sodium are safe, short-acting hypnotics with few adverse effects. They rarely cause hangover and are frequently used to treat insomnia in older patients. The prescribing guidelines applicable to BZD drugs should be followed when they are prescribed.

Barbiturates and paraldehyde are occasionally used to tranquillise patients who have not responded to other treatments or to treat status epilepticus. It is appropriate to consult an experienced colleague or the British National Formulary if considering prescribing these or other infrequently administered drugs.

Antihistamines, tricyclic AD drugs and low doses of typical and atypical antipsychotic drugs are also widely used for their hypnotic, sedative and anxiolytic properties. Meprobamate, invented over 60 years ago and hailed as the first tranquilliser (see Chapter 2) is still available for clinical use.

Antidepressant drugs as anxiolytic drugs

It has long been recognised that older AD drugs are effective in treating anxiety disorders. However, the adverse effects associated with these drugs militated against patients with anxiety taking them to an even greater extent than was the case with patients suffering from depression. This situation changed with the introduction of the SSRI AD drugs.

Several SSRI AD drugs appear to be as effective in treating anxiety disorders as older AD drugs but they cause fewer adverse effects and are therefore better tolerated by patients. The main difference between using SSRI and serotonin and noradrenaline (norepinephrine) reuptake inhibitor (SNRI) AD drugs to treat anxiety and using them to treat depression is that somewhat different dosages are required. Table 11.2 lists the anxiety disorders for which the SSRI and SNRI AD drugs are approved treatments currently available in the UK. Otherwise, the use of this group of drugs is similar in both groups of patients.

Table 11.2: The approved anxiety disorder indications, initial daily dose and daily dose range of the newer antidepressant drugs in the UK (dosing for the treatment of bulimia nervosa is also included)

AD drug	Anxiety disorder(s)	Initial daily dose[1]	Dose range[1]
Citalopram	Panic disorder	10 mg	20–60 mg
Escitalopram	Panic disorder	5 mg	10–20 mg
	Social phobia	5 mg	10–20 mg
Fluoxetine	Obsessive compulsive disorder	20 mg	20–60 mg
	Bulimia nervosa	60 mg	60 mg
Fluvoxamine	Obsessive compulsive disorder	50 mg	100–300 mg
Paroxetine[2]	Panic disorder	10 mg	20–60 mg
	Obsessive compulsive disorder	20 mg	20–60 mg
	Social phobia	20 mg	20–50 mg
	Post-traumatic stress disorder	20 mg	20–50 mg
	Generalised anxiety disorder	20 mg	20–50 mg
Sertraline	Obsessive compulsive disorder	50 mg	50–200 mg
	Post-traumatic stress disorder (women)	25 mg	50–200 mg
Venlafaxine[3]	Generalised anxiety disorder	75 mg	75 mg
Moclobemide	Social phobia	300 mg	600 mg

Notes:

[1]The above dosing recommendations refer only to the treatment of anxiety and bulimia nervosa. Dosing recommendations may differ when these drugs are used in the treatment of depression (see Chapter 9).

[2]The Committee on Safety of Medicines recommends 20 mg as the daily dose of paroxetine in the treatment of major depressive disorder, social phobia, generalised anxiety disorder and post-traumatic stress disorder and 40 mg as the daily dose of paroxetine in the treatment of obsessive-compulsive disorder and panic disorder on the grounds that there is no evidence that higher doses are more effective.

[3]The Committee on Safety of Medicines recommends that treatment with venlafaxine should be initiated and monitored by a specialist (including general practitioners with experience in psychiatry) because of concerns about cardiotoxicity and toxicity in overdose.

References and further reading

British National Formulary (2005) Available online at www.bnf.org.uk (accessed July 2005).

Committee on Safety of Medicines (1988) Benzodiazepines, dependence and withdrawal symptoms. Current Problems 21:1–2.

National Institute for Clinical Excellence (2004) Zaleplon, zolpidem and zopiclone for the short term management of insomnia. http://www.nice.org.uk/pdf/TA077 (accessed July 2005).

Petursson H, Lader MH (1981) Withdrawal from long term benzodiazepine treatment. British Medical Journal 283:643–645.

Zlotos DP (2005) Recent advances in melatonin receptor ligands. Archives of Pharmacology (Weinheim) 338(5–6):229–247.

12

Antiepileptic drugs

Introduction

Antiepileptic (AE) drugs are prescribed by neuropsychiatrists for the treatment of epilepsy and by general psychiatrists for the treatment of bipolar disorder. The AE drugs were invented and developed either as general sedatives or as specific treatments for epilepsy and their efficacy in bipolar disorder was discovered serendipitously.

This chapter provides an overview of the general pharmacological treatment of epilepsy. However, the reader is referred to a textbook of neurology for a more detailed treatment of this topic and of AE drugs. This overview will be followed by a detailed consideration of the AE drugs approved and/or widely prescribed in the UK for the treatment of bipolar disorder.

Antiepileptic drugs and epilepsy

The last decade has seen considerable advances in the treatment of epilepsy. These advances have been facilitated by:

- an improved understanding of the pathophysiology of epilepsy made possible by structural and functional neuroimaging and by computerised analysis of electroencephalographic (EEG) data and
- the invention and development of new AE drugs.

Pharmacodynamics of antiepileptic drugs

The principal mechanism of action of AE drugs involves enhancement of the neuroinhibitory effects of gamma-amino butyric acid (GABA). It will be recalled from Chapters 3 and 11 that benzodiazepine (BZD) drugs potentiate the neuroinhibitory effects of GABA (see Fig. 11.1). Briefly, binding of BZD drugs to the α subunit of the $GABA_A$ receptor alters the β subunit and facilitates its ability to bind GABA released from the presynaptic neurone. This in turn permits a greater influx of chloride ions and a greater degree of hyperpolarisation of the post-synaptic neurone than is possible through binding of GABA alone.

It is thought that the mechanism of action of carbamazepine, gabapentin, phenobarbital, phenytoin, primidone and topiramate is similar to that of BZD drugs. Carbamazepine also blocks N-methyl, D-aspartate (NMDA) receptors.

Sodium valproate, vigabatrin and tiagabine also promote GABA-ergic neuroinhibition. However, this effect is obtained via increased synaptic concentrations of GABA rather than by any direct effect at the GABA receptor. Thus sodium valproate stimulates GABA synthesis in the presynaptic neurone, vigabatrin inhibits GABA transaminase, the enzyme responsible for GABA degradation, and tiagabine inhibits the presynaptic reuptake transporter protein. Sodium valproate additionally causes upregulation of $GABA_B$ receptors.

Three drugs, carbamazepine, lamotrigine and topiramate, are glutamate antagonists that exert their AE effects by inhibiting glutamate-evoked postsynaptic depolarisation. Both achieve this by inhibiting glutamate (and aspartate) release at the synapse via blockade of presynaptic fast sodium channels. Topiramate is also an antagonist at non-NMDA glutamate receptors and a carbonic anhydrase inhibitor (and additionally has a mechanism of action similar to that of BZD drugs – see above).

Some aspects of the pharmacodynamics of the AE drugs that are widely prescribed in the treatment of acute mania and bipolar disorder – carbamazepine, lamotrigine and sodium valproate – are discussed further below.

Psychopharmacology and our understanding of epilepsy

The most widely accepted hypotheses about the aetiology of epileptic seizures are the inhibitory/excitatory neurotransmitter imbalance theory and the 'kindling' theory. The former postulates that an imbalance exists between inhibitory (predominantly GABA) and excitatory (predominantly glutamate) neurotransmitters that permits spontaneous excessive electrical activity in the brain which manifests as a seizure. This hypothesis derives from the probable mechanisms of action of AE drugs on GABE-ergic and glutamatergic systems as described above.

The 'kindling' theory is based on the finding that the repeated application of a sub-convulsive electrical stimulus to the brain will eventually cause a seizure when a further similar stimulus, or even a stimulus of a lesser magnitude, is applied. In patients with epilepsy, it is thought that recurrent discharges which do not cause a seizure 'kindle' the brain in such a manner that a further discharge of the same magnitude causes a seizure. It will be appreciated that AE drugs that enhance GABE-ergic and inhibit glutamatergic neurotransmission make the brain less susceptible to kindling.

General pharmacological treatment of epilepsy

The purpose of treating epilepsy is to prevent or greatly reduce the frequency of seizures by maintaining a therapeutic concentration of an AE drug or drugs in the brain.

The National Institute for Clinical Excellence recommends newer AE drugs such as gabapentin, lamotrigine, levetiracetam, oxcarbazepine, tiagabine, topiramate and vigabatrin, within their licensed indications, for the management of epilepsy in people who have not benefited from treatment with the older AE drugs or for whom the older AE drugs are unsuitable because of contraindications, interactions with other drugs including oral contraceptives, adverse effects or because the patient is a woman of childbearing potential (NICE, 2004).

Initiating treatment with antiepileptic drugs

Once initiated, treatment with AE drugs is likely to continue for many years and potentially throughout life. It is therefore imperative that such drugs are only prescribed following thorough observation and investigation of patients and a carefully considered diagnosis of epilepsy. It is not usual to initiate treatment with AE drugs following an initial epileptic seizure but it is recommended to do so following a second such seizure (NICE, 2004).

The choice of first-line AE drug depends on the predominant type of seizure experienced by the patient (see below). Treatment should be initiated at a relatively low dose which is then gradually titrated upwards until adequate control of seizures is obtained. If the initial AE drug that is prescribed (for example carbamazepine in the case of tonic/clonic seizures) is ineffective or causes unacceptable adverse effects, another appropriate first-line AE drug (for example lamotrigine in the case of tonic/clonic seizures) should be prescribed. This process should be continued until an AE drug proves effective or trials of treatment have been undertaken with all appropriate first-line AE drugs.

Monotherapy and combination therapy

If monotherapy is unsuccessful consideration must be given to combination therapy. The use of two or more AE drugs simultaneously, and in particular their pharmacokinetic interactions with each other (for example the induction of metabolic hepatic enzymes by carbamazepine increases the rate of metabolism and lowers plasma concentrations of lamotrigine and other AE drugs – see below), is now reasonably well understood. Nonetheless, two or more AE drugs should only be prescribed in combination when monotherapy with several appropriate AE drugs has proved ineffective or intolerable. NICE advise that 'combination therapy (adjunctive or 'add-on' therapy) should only be considered when attempts at monotherapy with AE drugs have not resulted in seizure freedom' (NICE, 2004).

Monitoring treatment with antiepileptic drugs

Therapeutic plasma concentrations have been determined for most AE drugs. However, with the exception of phenytoin, measuring such plasma concentrations is of little value because the purpose of prescribing an AE drug is to treat an individual patient with epilepsy rather than maintain the plasma level of a drug within an arbitrary range. Thus if seizures are controlled and a patient is not experiencing adverse effects, plasma levels above the therapeutic range can probably be ignored. Conversely, if levels are within the therapeutic range but seizures continue, dosage may be increased until efficacy is achieved or until adverse effects occur. Equally, dosage should not be increased if it is effective, despite plasma levels below the therapeutic range.

NICE advises that monitoring the plasma levels of AE drugs 'should be done only if clinically indicated' and particularly in order to:

- detect non-adherence to prescribed medication
- manage suspected toxicity
- adjust phenytoin dose (the metabolism of phenytoin is saturable and a modest increase in dose may cause a dramatic increase in plasma concentration and lead to toxicity)
- manage drug/drug interactions between AE drugs prescribed in combination and
- manage clinical conditions, for example status epilepticus, organ failure and pregnancy (NICE, 2004).

The risk of interactions between AE drugs is high and some interactions are unpredictable. The mechanism of such interactions may be either hepatic enzyme induction or hepatic enzyme inhibition. The effects of AE drug/drug interactions on the plasma concentrations of the most commonly prescribed AE drugs is presented in Table 12.1. It is worth noting that these effects may be mediated through increased or reduced plasma concentrations of active metabolites of the parent

Table 12.1: Antiepileptic drug/drug interactions and their effect on plasma concentrations of the most commonly prescribed antiepileptic drugs

Antiepileptic drug	Increased plasma concentration	Reduced plasma concentration
Carbamazepine	Phenytoin	Carbamazepine (see below), clobazam, clonazepam, lamotrigine, phenytoin, tiagabine, topiramate, sodium valproate
Ethosuximide	Phenytoin	–
Gabapentin	–	–
Lamotrigine	–	–
Levetiracetam	–	–
Oxcarbazepine	Phenytoin, phenobarbital	Carbamazepine
Phenobarbital and primidone	–	Carbamazepine, clonazepam, ethosuximide, lamotrigine, tiagabine, topiramate, sodium valproate
Phenytoin	Phenobarbital	Carbamazepine, clonazepam, ethosuximide, lamotrigine, tiagabine, topiramate, sodium valproate
Pregabalin	–	–
Tiagabine	–	Sodium valproate
Topiramate	Phenytoin	–
Sodium valproate	Carbamazepine, ethosuximide, lamotrigine, primidone, phenobarbital, phenytoin, primidone	–
Vigabatrin	–	Phenobarbital, phenytoin, primidone

AE drug. Monitoring plasma concentrations may be helpful when two or more AE drugs are prescribed in combination, particularly while patients are being established on effective doses.

AE drugs may increase or reduce plasma concentrations of non-AE drugs and, conversely, non-AE drugs may increase or reduce plasma concentrations of AE drugs. It is therefore essential to consider drug/ drug interactions when prescribing an AE drug for a patient who is already taking a non-AE drug or when prescribing a non-AE drug for a patient who is already taking an AE drug.

Contraception and reproduction

AE drugs including carbamazepine, lamotrigine, phenobarbital, phenytoin and topiramate induce the metabolism of ethinyloestradiol and impair the efficacy of the combined hormonal contraceptive pill. The risk of unwanted pregnancy may be reduced by two methods:

1. Use of an alternative method of contraception such as a parenteral progesterone-only contraceptive (in which case the injection interval should be reduced from 12 to 10 weeks) or an intrauterine contraceptive device. Neither orally administered nor implantable progesterone-only contraceptives are regarded as reliable in women taking enzyme-inducing AE drugs.

2. Prescription of a combination contraceptive pill (or combination of pills) containing a dosage of at least 50 micrograms ethinyloestradiol daily. If breakthrough bleeding continues it is appropriate to increase the dosage of ethinyloestradiol to 100 micrograms daily.

In the event that neither of the above options is suitable or effective, the prescription of an AE drug that does not induce hepatic enzymes such as gabapentin, sodium valproate or vigabatrin should be considered.

Women with epilepsy should plan their pregnancies and should consider withdrawing AE drugs both before conception and during pregnancy. This decision must be taken carefully however, because it is almost certainly safer to take AE drugs while pregnant than to experience seizures. Carbamazepine is probably the least teratogenic AE drug. Folate supplements are advised for women taking AE drugs (and are now advised for all women), both before and during pregnancy. Vitamin K supplements are additionally advised for pregnant women taking carbamazepine, phenobarbital or phenytoin, because of the risk of neonatal bleeding.

Adverse effects of antiepileptic drugs

The specific adverse effects of individual AE drugs are considered below. Three general adverse effects of AE drugs warrant mention as follows:

1. AE drugs that induce hepatic enzymes increase the rate of metabolism of vitamin D and patients at risk of vitamin D deficiency (pregnant women or individuals who are malnourished, for example) may develop osteomalacia or rickets. Vitamin D supplementation may therefore be necessary.

2. Most AE drugs have a negative and dose-dependent effect on cognitive function. This is most evident for benzodiazepine and barbiturate AE drugs and least evident for gabapentin, lamotrigine and vigabatrin. Carbamazepine, phenytoin, sodium valproate and topiramate pose an intermediate risk.

3. Some epileptic patients who have been effectively treated with AE drugs may experience depression, mania and/or psychotic symptoms in association with a reduction in seizures and normalisation of their EEG. This syndrome, which has been referred to as alternative psychosis or forced normalisation, has also been reported following the neurosurgical treatment of epilepsy. It may often be alleviated by a slight reduction in AE drug dosage such that the EEG exhibits some epileptic activity and/or occasional seizures occur.

Discontinuation of antiepileptic drugs

Patients who have not experienced seizures for a prolonged period may understandably wish to discontinue their AE drugs. Any decision to do this must be individualised and take account of the following factors:

- The type of epilepsy the patient suffers with. Absence seizures tend to remit spontaneously during adolescence and it may be appropriate to continue AE drug treatment and await this. On the other hand seizures almost always reoccur in patients with juvenile myoclonic epilepsy when AE drugs are withdrawn.

- The presence of structural brain abnormality demonstrated by EEG or neuroimaging or by the presence of neurological signs on clinical examination. It is often difficult to control seizures in patients with structural brain abnormality and there is a significant risk of recurrence of seizures if AE drugs are withdrawn.

- The length of time the patient has been free of seizures. A 2-year minimum is recommended.

- The normality of the EEG with current AE drug treatment. It would be unwise to withdraw treatment from a patient whose EEG continues to exhibit significant epileptic activity despite treatment with AE drugs.

- Any adverse effects of current AE drug treatment.

- Social factors such as the patient's occupation, domestic situation and leisure pursuits.

- The patient's need for a driving licence. Many patients with epilepsy hold a driving licence because they meet the requirements of the Driver and Vehicle Licensing Agency and have either not experienced any seizures for at least 1 year or have experienced seizures only while asleep for at least 3 years. Such patients must not drive while their AE drugs are being withdrawn and for at least 6 months following such withdrawal and must be advised that reoccurrence of seizures means the loss of a driving licence.

If it is decided to withdraw AE drugs this must be undertaken gradually over a period of 3 to 6 months because abrupt withdrawal, particularly of benzodiazepine or barbiturate drugs, may cause seizures. A careful record of seizure type and frequency should be made and an EEG recorded before reducing dosage, again when dosage is reduced to approximately half the initial dosage, and finally when AE drugs are discontinued. Any increase in seizure frequency or severity, or deterioration in the EEG, should lead to the planned withdrawal being reconsidered, deferred or abandoned.

Patients receiving a combination of AE drugs should be withdrawn from one drug at a time and should be monitored carefully following such withdrawal for a period of 3 to 6 months before withdrawal of a further AE drug is considered.

Approximately 60% of carefully selected patients remain seizure free following AE drug withdrawal.

Generalised epilepsy

Patients who experience seizures most often require treatment for either generalised epilepsy or for partial or focal epilepsy.

Patients with generalised epilepsy exhibit abnormal electrical activity throughout the brain during a seizure. They always experience impairment of consciousness. In addition they may experience tonic/ clonic, absence, myoclonic or atypical seizures. The choice of AE drugs for the first-line monotherapy treatment of generalised epilepsy depends on which of these types of seizure are predominantly experienced by the patient.

Tonic/clonic seizures

Tonic/clonic (or grand mal) seizures respond best to carbamazepine, lamotrigine, phenytoin or sodium valproate. Barbiturates such as phenobarbital are also effective but their adverse effects, particularly sedation and cognitive impairment, mean that they have a limited place in the contemporary treatment of tonic/clonic epilepsy.

Absence seizures

Absence (or petit mal) seizures respond best to ethosuximide or sodium valproate. Many patients with epilepsy experience both tonic/clonic and absence seizures. Sodium valproate is an effective treatment for such patients. Lamotrigine is also effective although it is not currently approved for this indication in the UK.

Myoclonic seizures

Myoclonic seizures may respond to clonazepam, ethosuximide, lamotrigine or sodium valproate. Some patients gain further benefit from the addition of piracetam, whose mechanism of action is not understood, to one or other of these AE drugs.

Atypical seizures

Atypical seizures include atypical absence seizures as well as atonic and tonic seizures. They are difficult to treat but may respond to clonazepam, ethosuximide, lamotrigine, phenytoin or sodium valproate. Phenobarbital or acetazolamide may be useful if these prove ineffective.

Partial or focal epilepsy

Patients with partial or focal epilepsy exhibit abnormal electrical activity in a specific region of the brain during a seizure. This causes motor, sensory and/or neuropsychiatric symptoms. Whether they experience impaired consciousness (partial complex epilepsy) or not (partial simple epilepsy) depends on whether or not the abnormal electrical activity spreads. Partial or focal seizures that spread to cause abnormal electrical activity throughout the brain produce tonic/clonic seizures referred to as secondary generalised seizures.

The recommended first-line monotherapy AE drugs for partial or focal epilepsy are carbamazepine, lamotrigine, phenytoin and valproate. If none of these drugs are effective two of them may be prescribed in combination. Alternatively, a drug such as acetazolamide, clobazam, clonazepam, gabapentin, tiagabine, topiramate or vigabatrin may be added to the most effective monotherapy identified from carbamazepine, lamotrigine, phenytoin and valproate. Barbiturates have little place in the contemporary treatment of partial or focal epilepsy for the reasons stated above.

Status epilepticus

Status epilepticus consists of recurrent seizures that occur without recovery of consciousness between them and that persist for at least 30 minutes. Guidance on the treatment of status epilepticus has recently been provided by NICE (2004).

Patients with status epilepticus may need resuscitation, intubation and/or ventilation and are best treated in an intensive care unit. Treatment requires immediate intravenous (IV) lorazepam in a dose of 0.1 mg per kg bodyweight administered at a rate of 2 mg per minute. IV diazepam in a dose of 10 to 20 mg administered at a rate of 5 mg per minute may also be used (as may midazolam and clonazepam). However, IV lorazepam is preferred to IV diazepam because it has a longer duration of antiepileptic action. Paraldehyde administered rectally is sometimes used while anaesthesia with thiopentone or propofol may occasionally be required. In addition to controlling seizures it is important that any presumed cause of status epilepticus, for example thiamine deficiency in alcohol-dependent patients, is also treated.

The acute treatment of status epilepticus should be followed by an IV infusion of phenytoin in a dose of 15 mg per kg bodyweight administered at a rate of 50 mg per minute. Alternatively, an IV infusion of fosphenytoin in a dose of 15 mg per kg bodyweight may be administered at a rate of 100 to 150 mg per minute. Fosphenytoin is a pro-drug that is metabolised to phenytoin following administration.

Psychotropic drugs and epilepsy

Given the prevalence of epilepsy and psychiatric illness, the occurrence of both in an individual patient is not at all uncommon. This presents a clinical problem because both antidepressant (AD) and antipsychotic (AP) drugs increase the risk of seizures developing or being exacerbated.

Tricyclic AD drugs are significantly more likely to cause seizures than selective serotonin reuptake inhibitor (SSRI) AD drugs. The latter therefore represent the AD drugs of choice in depressed patients with epilepsy. If an SSRI is not effective or is not tolerated in such a patient, monoamine oxidase inhibitor AD drugs, which have slight anticonvulsant properties, may be appropriate.

Patients treated with high doses of chlorpromazine have a 10% risk for developing seizures while for other AP drugs the risk is below 1%. Of the atypical AP drugs, risperidone poses the least risk and clozapine the greatest, with olanzapine and quetiapine posing an intermediate risk. The occurrence of seizures in 5629 patients treated with clozapine has been reviewed by Pacia and Devinsky (1994). The frequency of tonic/clonic seizures was 1.3%. Seizures occurred at doses below 300 mg daily during the titration phase of treatment and at doses above 600 mg daily during the maintenance phase. Of patients who experienced seizures, 78% of those who were rechallenged were able to continue treatment with clozapine following very gradual dose titration and, in some cases, the addition of AE drugs. This finding supports the view that concern about the epileptogenic effect of AP drugs should not prevent the treatment of psychosis in patients with a history of seizures or a diagnosis of epilepsy (Mitchell, 2004). Even if seizures reoccur or are exacerbated, AE drugs can be commenced or their dose may be increased.

Antiepileptic drugs and bipolar disorder

Three AE drugs – carbamazepine, lamotrigine and both sodium valproate and valproate semisodium – are widely prescribed for the treatment of acute mania and for prophylaxis in bipolar disorder and their use in this regard has been described in Chapter 10. Their pharmacology will now be considered.

The pharmacodynamics of AE drugs have been discussed above while the somewhat modest contribution of psychopharmacology to our understanding of bipolar disorder has been considered in Chapter 10.

Carbamazepine

Carbamazepine is a dibenzazepine derivative that is approved in the UK for the prophylaxis of manic-depressive psychosis in patients unresponsive to lithium therapy.

Pharmacokinetics

Carbamazepine is absorbed relatively slowly and only reaches C_{MAX} in 6–12 hours. Plasma protein binding is high at approximately 85% while its $T_{1/2}$ varies from 50 hours when initially administered to 5 hours following chronic administration. This reduction in $T_{1/2}$ occurs because carbamazepine is metabolised by cytochrome 3A4 enzymes and induces its own metabolic enzymes. These enzymes also reduce blood levels of lamotrigine, valproate, AP drugs, barbiturates, clobazam, clonazepam, ethinyloestradiol (see advice on contraception above), ethosuximide, phenytoin, tricyclic AD drugs, tiagabine, topiramate and warfarin. Carbamazepine does not inhibit metabolic enzymes.

Efficacy

The various uses of carbamazepine in patients with epilepsy have already been noted. Carbamazepine may also be prescribed as:

- an antimanic drug in the treatment of acute mania and as
- a mood stabiliser in the prophylaxis of bipolar disorder in patients unresponsive to or intolerant of lithium. In this case it may be prescribed alone or, more often, in combination with lithium.

Evidence for the efficacy of carbamazepine as an antimanic drug is limited and such use is not approved in the UK. Evidence of efficacy as a mood stabilising drug is less convincing than that for lithium, valproate, olanzapine and lamotrigine and its use in this context has declined in recent years.

Treatment with carbamazepine should be commenced at 200 mg twice daily and increased by 200 mg per day every 2–3 weeks. Patients with mania may require doses of up to 1600 mg daily while a dose in the range 400–600 mg daily is usually adequate for prophylaxis. Plasma carbamazepine levels of 4–12 mg/l are recommended but these are of very limited value and clinical status is the best determinant of a patient's optimal dose (see above).

Safety

Nausea, headache, dizziness, ataxia, diplopia and confusion are the commonest adverse effects of carbamazepine. Less common but more serious adverse effects are as follows:

* An itchy erythematous rash, the risk of which may be reduced by slow titration of dose. Carbamazepine must be withdrawn if this rash is significant or if it occurs in association with fever and/or haematological abnormalities (leucopaenia, thrombocytopaenia). Clinical chemistry and haematological parameters should be evaluated before and during the first month of treatment.
* Stevens–Johnson syndrome, toxic epidermal necrolysis.
* Agranulocytosis, aplastic anaemia, lymphadenopathy.
* Cholestatic jaundice, hepatitis, acute renal failure, hyponatraemia, oedema, osteomalacia.
* Gynaecomastia, galactorrhoea, impotence.
* Dyskinesia, psychosis, depression, aggression.

Carbamazepine is teratogenic and may cause neural tube defects if taken during pregnancy. Women should discontinue treatment with it 3 months prior to conception and should not take it during pregnancy. They should take folate supplements both pre-conceptually and during pregnancy. Such supplements are particularly vital if carbamazepine must be continued during pregnancy, a not infrequent clinical situation given that it is probably the least teratogenic of the currently available AE drugs (Morrow et al, 2005).

Carbamazepine is structurally related to tricyclic AD drugs and should not be prescribed simultaneously or within 2 weeks of treatment with monoamine oxidase inhibitor AD drugs.

Lamotrigine

Lamotrigine is a phenyltriazine that is not currently approved for administration to patients with bipolar disorder in the UK. Nonetheless, it is commonly prescribed for such patients.

Pharmacokinetics

Lamotrigine is absorbed rapidly and reaches C_{MAX} in 2.5 hours. It has a $T_{1/2}$ of approximately 30 hours. Plasma protein binding is modest at approximately 55%. Lamotrigine induces metabolic enzymes.

Efficacy

The various uses of lamotrigine in patients with epilepsy have already been noted. Lamotrigine was noted to elevate mood in patients with epilepsy and this led to clinical trials in which lamotrigine was investigated as:

* an adjuvant with paroxetine in major depressive disorder (Normann et al, 2002)
* an adjuvant with fluoxetine in treatment-resistant major depressive disorder (Barbosa et al, 2003)
* an AD drug in the treatment of bipolar depressive disorder (Calabrese et al, 1999) and
* a mood stabiliser in the prophylaxis of bipolar disorder.

Lamotrigine is approved in the US as a mood stabiliser in the prophylaxis of bipolar disorder. It is particularly effective in patients with bipolar disorder who experience predominantly recurrent depressive episodes. Lamotrigine does not seem to be an effective antimanic drug and is probably not an effective mood stabiliser in the prophylaxis of bipolar disorder in patients who experience predominantly manic or mixed relapses.

Treatment with lamotrigine should be commenced at 25 mg daily for 2 weeks and increased slowly (by 25–50 mg per day) every 2–3 weeks. The usual maximum dose is 100–250 mg daily. The dose of lamotrigine should be reduced in patients who are also taking sodium valproate. Clinical status is the best determinant of a patient's optimal dose.

Safety

Vomiting, dizziness, drowsiness, headache, diplopia, ataxia and confusion are the most common adverse effects. About 10% of patients develop a rash and slow titration of dose helps to minimise this risk. Any rash must be monitored extremely carefully because it may progress to Stevens–Johnson syndrome and toxic epidermal necrolysis. An influenza-like syndrome may also occur. Patients should be advised to seek medical attention immediately if a rash or influenza-like syndrome develops. Very rare cases of status epilepticus, multiple organ failure and death have been reported when lamotrigine is administered in combination with other AE drugs.

Sodium valproate

Sodium valproate is a branched chain fatty acid that is not currently approved for administration to patients with bipolar disorder in the UK (see valproate semisodium below). Nonetheless, like lamotrigine, it is commonly prescribed for such patients.

Pharmacokinetics

Sodium valproate is readily absorbed and reaches C_{MAX} in approximately 6 hours. It undergoes rapid hepatic metabolism. Plasma protein binding is approximately 90% while $T_{1/2}$ is 8–10 hours. Sodium valproate does not induce metabolic enzymes but it inhibits enzymes that metabolise carbamazepine, ethosuximide, lamotrigine, phenobarbital, phenytoin and primidone and causes their plasma levels to increase.

Efficacy

The various uses of sodium valproate in patients with epilepsy have already been noted. Sodium valproate is also frequently prescribed as:

- an antimanic drug in the treatment of acute mania and
- a mood stabiliser in the prophylaxis of bipolar disorder in patients unresponsive to or intolerant of lithium. In this case it may be prescribed alone or in combination with lithium.

Treatment with sodium valproate should be commenced at 200 mg twice daily and increased by 200 mg per day every 2–3 days. Patients with mania may require doses of up to 2000 mg daily while 1000 to 2000 mg daily is usually adequate for prophylaxis. Plasma valproate levels of 50–150 mg/l are recommended but these are of limited value and clinical status is the best determinant of a patient's optimal dose.

Safety

Nausea, ataxia, tremor, weight gain (which may be marked) and reversible hair loss (although regrown hair may be curly) are the commonest adverse effects of sodium valproate. They occur less frequently with slow-release preparations. Less common but more serious adverse effects include:

- Hepatotoxicity which may be severe, and occasionally fatal, in children and in patients taking other AE drugs in addition to sodium valproate. Liver function should be evaluated before commencing treatment, and during the first 6 months of treatment. Impending hepatotoxicity may be marked by malaise, anorexia, drowsiness and abdominal pain and, in patients with epilepsy, the return of or exacerbation of seizures.
- Stevens–Johnson syndrome.
- Pancreatitis.
- Hyperammonaemia with confusion and asterixis (clinical chemistry parameters should be monitored).
- Blood dyscrasias including leucopaenia and pancytopaenia (haematological parameters should be monitored).

Sodium valproate is teratogenic and may cause congenital cardiac defects and neonatal seizures if taken during pregnancy.

Valproate semisodium

Valproate semisodium, a dimer composed of two sodium valproate molecules, is approved in the UK for the acute treatment of manic episodes associated with bipolar disorder.

Treatment with valproate semisodium should be commenced at 250 mg twice daily and increased by 250 mg per day every 2–3 days. Patients with mania may require doses of up to 2250 mg daily while 1250–2250 mg daily is usually adequate for prophylaxis. Clinical status is the best determinant of a patient's optimal dose.

Other antiepileptic drugs

A number of other AE drugs, most notably gabapentin, phenytoin, topiramate and vigabatrin are occasionally employed in the treatment of patients with bipolar disorder. None of these are approved for such use and evidence for their efficacy in bipolar disorder is absent or modest. Their use must therefore be regarded as experimental at present.

References and further reading

Barbosa L, Berk M, Vorster M (2003) A double-blind, randomized, placebo-controlled trial of augmentation with lamotrigine or placebo in patients concomitantly treated with fluoxetine for resistant major depressive episodes. Journal of Clinical Psychiatry 64(4):403–407.

Calabrese JR, Bowden CL, Sachs GS, Ascher JA, Monaghan E, Rudd GD (1999) A double-blind placebo-controlled study of lamotrigine monotherapy in outpatients with bipolar I depression. Lamictal 602 Study Group. Journal of Clinical Psychiatry 60(2):79–88.

Driver and Vehicle Licensing Agency. www.dvla.gov.uk (accessed July 2005).

Mackin P, Young A (2004) Bipolar disorders. In: Core Psychiatry (Eds Wright P, Phelan M and Stern J) (2nd Edition). London, Elsevier Saunders, pp. 295–318.

Mitchell AJ (2004) Epilepsy. In: Neuropsychiatry and behavioural neurology explained (Mitchell AJ). Saunders, Edinburgh, pp. 113–126.

Morrow JI, Russell A, Guthrie (2005) Malformation risks of antiepileptic drugs in pregnancy: a prospective study from the UK Epilepsy and Pregnancy Register. Journal of Neurology, Neurosurgery and Psychiatry 77:193–198.

National Institute for Clinical Excellence (2004) The epilepsies: the diagnosis and management of the epilepsies in adults and children in primary and secondary care (www.nice.org.uk) (accessed July 2005).

Normann C, Hummel B, Scharer LO, Horn M, Grunze H, Walden J (2002) Lamotrigine as adjunct to paroxetine in acute depression: a placebo-controlled, double-blind study. Journal of Clinical Psychiatry 63(4):337–344.

Pacia SV, Devinsky O (1994) Clozapine-related seizures: experience with 5629 patients. Neurology 44(12):2247–2249.

Wright P, Sigmundsson T (2004) Organic psychiatry and epilepsy. In: Core Psychiatry (Eds Wright P, Phelan M and Stern J) (2nd Edition). London, Elsevier Saunders, pp. 381–411.

13

Sexual disorders

Introduction

Drugs currently have a more significant role to play in the treatment of sexual disorders in men than in women. The phosphodiesterase type 5 (PDE-5) inhibitors have revolutionised the treatment of erectile dysfunction and drugs also have a place in the treatment of premature ejaculation and in the management of male antisocial sexual behaviour.

There are as yet no drugs approved in the UK, or indeed anywhere, for the treatment of female sexual dysfunction. A few approved for other purposes are of value and new drugs specifically designed to treat female sexual dysfunction are being developed. One benefit of hormone replacement therapy following menopause is the prevention of female sexual dysfunction and the reader is referred to a textbook of medicine or gynaecology for a more detailed treatment of this topic.

Erectile dysfunction

Drugs used in the treatment of erectile dysfunction (ED) may be divided into:

1. Newer drugs, the phosphodiesterase type 5 (PDE-5) inhibitors, which are administered orally and which have largely supplanted the older drugs.
2. Older drugs, many of which are administered by intracavernosal injection.

Phosphodiesterase type 5 inhibitors

The PDE-5 inhibitors include sildenafil, tadalafil and vardenafil. Sildenafil, the first PDE5 inhibitor to be discovered, was originally investigated in male patients with angina in whom it was serendipitously observed to improve erectile function. All three drugs are potent and, most importantly, highly selective inhibitors of PDE5 when administered orally (see Table 13.1).

Pharmacokinetics

The available PDE-5 inhibitors differ from each other pharmacokinetically and these differences have clinical implications (see below). Sildenafil is rapidly absorbed and reaches C_{MAX} in 1 hour. Plasma protein binding is in excess of 95%. Metabolism via hepatic microsomal enzymes, predominantly CYP3A4, produces a clinically active major metabolite, N-desmethyl sildenafil. Sildenafil has a $T_{1/2}$ of approximately 4 hours.

Tadalafil is rapidly absorbed and reaches C_{MAX} in 2 hours. Plasma protein binding is in excess of 95%. Metabolism via hepatic microsomal enzymes, predominantly CYP3A4, produces a clinically inactive major metabolite. Tadalafil has a $T_{1/2}$ of approximately 15 hours.

Vardenafil is rapidly absorbed and reaches C_{MAX} in 1 hour. Plasma protein binding is in excess of 95%. Metabolism via hepatic microsomal enzymes, predominantly CYP3A4, produces a clinically active major metabolite, desethyl vardenafil. Vardenafil has a $T_{1/2}$ of approximately 4 hours.

Pharmacodynamics

The enzyme nitric oxide synthetase in the endothelial cells of the corpus cavernosum converts L-arginine to nitric oxide (NO) and L-citrulline. Penile erection depends upon the release of NO from these endothelial cells in response to psychological or physical stimulation (Fig. 13.1). NO binds to guanylate (or guanylyl) cyclase and activates it and guanylyl cyclase in turn catalyses the conversion of 5-guanosine triphosphate (GTP) to 3,5-cyclic guanosine monophosphate (cGMP) and pyrophosphate. Protein kinase is activated by cGMP and in turn phosphorylates contractile proteins and reduces calcium concentrations, thus inhibiting contraction of smooth muscle. Increased concentrations of cGMP therefore cause relaxation of smooth muscle in the arteries and trabeculae of the corpus callosum. These changes permit erection by both increased perfusion of the penis and sustained distension of the cavernosal spaces with blood.

PDE-5, or more correctly cGMP specific PDE-5, is the enzyme responsible for degrading cGMP to 5-guanosine monophosphate (GMP) in the penis. PDE-5 inhibitors therefore facilitate erection by

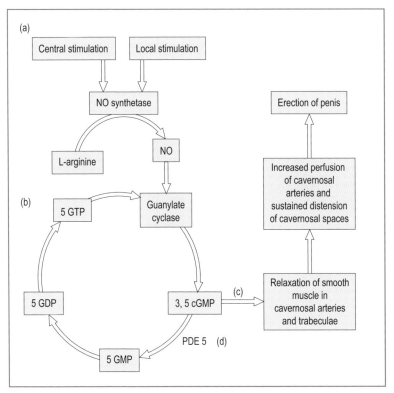

Fig. 13.1 Role of nitric oxide and phosphodiesterase type 5 in penile physiology. (**a**) Central psychological and/or local physical stimulation activates nitric oxide synthetase in the endothelial cells of the corpus cavernosum. Nitric oxide synthetase catalyses the conversion of L-arginine to nitric oxide (NO) which in turn activates guanylate cyclase. (**b**) Guanylate cyclase catalyses the conversion of 5-guanosine triphosphate (5-GTP) to 3,5-cyclic guanosine monophosphate (3,5-cGMP). (**c**) 3,5-cGMP activates protein kinase in smooth muscle in the arteries and trabeculae of the corpus callosum. Protein kinase phosphorylates contractile proteins and reduces calcium concentrations, thus inhibiting smooth muscle contraction and causing dilatation of cavernosal arteries and spaces. These changes permit erection by both increased vascular perfusion of the penis and sustained distension of the cavernosal spaces with blood. (**d**) Erection does not occur in the absence of central or local stimulation because while 3,5-cGMP is produced, it is rapidly metabolised by phosphodiesterase type 5 (PDE-5) to 5-GMP and thence to 5-guanosine diphosphate (5-GDP) and 5-GTP.

preventing the degradation of cGMP (Fig. 13.2). It is important to appreciate that this mechanism of action permits erection only in response to psychological or physical stimulation and does not cause erection independently of such stimulation.

Eleven different PDE enzymes have been identified in the human body. Sildenafil, tadalafil and vardenefil have high affinity for PDE-5

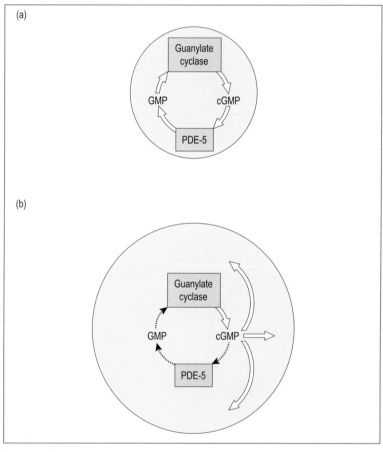

Fig. 13.2 Role of phosphodiesterase type 5 inhibitors in the treatment of erectile dysfunction. (**a**) Psychological and/or physical stimulation does lead to the production of nitric oxide (NO) and cyclic guanosine monophosphate (cGMP) in men with erectile dysfunction. However, insufficient quantities of cGMP are available to permit erection. (**b**) Phosphodiesterase type 5 inhibitors block the first metabolic step in the degradation of cGMP. This ensures that sufficient quantities of cGMP are available to permit erection (indicated by the enlarged circle) in response to psychological and/or physical stimulation.

which occurs primarily in the penis. They have almost no affinity for other PDE enzymes and hence almost no enzyme inhibiting effect at sites other than the penis.

Efficacy

The three PDE5 inhibitors are effective in approximately 70% of patients with erectile dysfunction. Tadalafil may be taken 0.5–12 hours before anticipated sexual activity and remains effective for 24 hours or more (hence the sobriquet 'le weekender'). Sildenafil and vardenafil must be taken no more than 1 hour before anticipated sexual activity. They have a shorter duration of effect than tadalafil.

The PDE5 inhibitors are occasionally prescribed for the treatment of sexual dysfunction associated with long-term use of selective serotonin reuptake inhibitor (SSRI) antidepressant (AD) drugs.

Safety

PDE5 inhibitors should not be administered concomitantly with:

- nitrates or NO donors such as amyl nitrate or
- potent inhibitors of CYP3A4 including the protease inhibitor, ritonavir, and the antifungal agents, ketoconazole and itraconazole.

The common adverse effects of PDE5 inhibitors include headache, dizziness, nasal congestion, flushing, dyspepsia, nausea, rhinitis and sinusitis. Sudden visual loss due to non-arteritic anterior ischaemic optic neuropathy has been reported but it is currently unclear if this is caused by PDE5 inhibitors or by comorbid disease, for example diabetes mellitus. Patients taking PDE5 inhibitors should be advised to seek immediate medical care if they experience visual loss. Abnormal colour vision has been reported with sildenafil. Priapism may occur, especially in patients with sickle-cell anaemia, multiple myeloma or leukaemia. PDE5 inhibitors should be used cautiously if the penis is anatomically deformed, for example by Peyronie's disease.

Table 13.1: The initial daily dose, daily dose range and available formulations of the prostaglandin type 5 inhibitors

PDE5 inhibitor	Initial dose	Dose range	Available formulations
Sildenafil	50 mg	25–100 mg	Tablets
Tadalafil	10 mg	10–20 mg	Tablets
Vardenafil	10 mg	5–20 mg	Tablets

Older drugs

Older drugs for the treatment of erectile impotence have been largely replaced by the PDE5 inhibitors. Nonetheless, they are relatively effective and may be appropriate for patients in whom PDE5 inhibitors are either contraindicated or are ineffective. The most effective of the older drugs are:

- Papaverine – this smooth muscle relaxant may be effective alone or in combination with phentolamine (see below). It is administered by intracavernosal injection.
- Phentolamine – this short-acting α_1 noradrenergic receptor antagonist is usually administered in combination with papaverine by intracavernosal injection. Phenoxybenzamine, a long-acting α_1 noradrenergic receptor antagonist, is no longer used.
- Alprostadil – this naturally occurring form of prostaglandin E_1 may be administered by intracavernosal injection or intraurethral insertion. It induces erection by relaxation of trabecular smooth muscle in the corpus cavernosum and dilation of cavernosal arteries.

Although relatively effective, the use of these drugs is limited because of:

- administration by uncomfortable intracavernosal injection or intraurethral insertion
- onset of erection following administration and independently of sexual stimulation and
- the need to complete sexual activity within approximately one hour of administration.

The most troublesome adverse effect of older drugs is priapism. This may require urgent aspiration of the corpus cavernosum, intracavernosal injection of phenylephrine or adrenaline (epinephrine), or surgery.

Older orally administered drugs for erectile dysfunction include apomorphine and yohimbine. Apomorphine is a centrally acting dopamine (DA) receptor agonist that has relative specificity for DA D_2 receptors. Stimulation of these receptors in the hypothalamus promotes the transport of oxytocin from the hypothalamus to the posterior pituitary gland from which it enters the systemic circulation. Oxytocin signalling promotes NO synthesis at the penis. Yohimbine is an α_2 noradrenergic receptor antagonist. The use of these drugs has declined with the advent of the PDE5 inhibitors.

Premature ejaculation

SSRI AD drugs cause delayed ejaculation in a proportion of patients to whom they are administered for the treatment of depression. Although not an approved indication, this adverse effect has been used to advantage in the treatment of premature ejaculation.

Antisocial sexual behaviour

Cyproterone acetate and benperidol may be prescribed in an attempt to reduce libido and control antisocial sexual behaviour in men. Medroxyprogesterone and the luteinising hormone analogue, goserelin, are prescribed less frequently for this purpose. Fully informed consent and the completion of certain legal requirements are a necessary prerequisite to such treatment. Prescribing is best initiated and monitored by a clinician experienced in the use of antiandrogenic treatment in the management of antisocial sexual behaviour.

Cyproterone acetate has a dual mechanism of action. Testosterone and other androgens influence regions of the brain that play an essential role in male sexual drive. Cyproterone acetate reduces the effect of testosterone and other androgens on these regions by blockade of androgen receptors. It also has a progestogenic effect which inhibits the release of gonadotrophins from the hypothalamus. This, in turn, inhibits the release of androgens from the testicles. Cyproterone acetate has relatively few adverse effects and its action is completely reversible.

Benperidol is a butyrophenone drug with a similar mechanism of action and adverse effect profile to haloperidol (see Chapter 8). It is approved in the UK for the 'control of deviant antisocial sexual behaviour' and should be prescribed in a dose of 0.25 to 1.5 mg daily.

Female sexual dysfunction

There are no drugs available at present specifically for the treatment of female sexual dysfunction. Hormone replacement therapy, primarily prescribed for the prevention of osteoporosis in post-menopausal women, provides an additional benefit to many women in that it helps maintain sexual function by preventing loss of libido and by slowing age-related changes in the genitalia (see above). Topically applied oestrogen cream may also be helpful in the treatment of age-related changes in the genitalia.

The PDE5 inhibitors have been investigated in female sexual dysfunction and found to be of benefit to some women with sexual arousal disorder and in whom libido is normal but genital engorgement does not occur in response to psychological or physical stimulation. They are therefore occasionally prescribed for such women on the grounds that they increase perfusion of the female genitalia. Testosterone is prescribed very occasionally for women with the intent of increasing libido.

Experimental drugs for the treatment of female sexual dysfunction include:

- PGE1 such as alprostadil (see above) intended to treat sexual arousal disorder by increasing perfusion of the genitalia
- α_1 noradrenergic receptor antagonists intended to treat sexual arousal disorder by increasing perfusion of the genitalia and
- testosterone and testosterone analogues intended to treat impaired libido.

References and further reading

British National Formulary (2004) British Medical Association and Royal Pharmaceutical Society of Great Britain. London (www.bnf.org).

Cookson J, Taylor D, Katona C (2002) Use of Drugs in Psychiatry. Gaskell, London.

14

Alcohol, drug and nicotine misuse

Introduction

Misuse of, and dependence upon, alcohol and psychotropic drugs, including nicotine, represents a major problem for individuals and for society. Significant advances have been made in our understanding of the psychopharmacology of misuse and dependence in recent years. Advances have also been made in the psychopharmacological treatment of alcohol and drug misuse.

This chapter will summarise our current understanding of the psychopharmacology of alcohol, drug and nicotine misuse. The psychotropic drugs currently available for the treatment of such misuse will then be considered.

The psychopharmacology of alcohol, drug and nicotine misuse

Research during the last 25 years has revealed that the experience of pleasure is largely mediated by increased release of dopamine (DA) at the nucleus accumbens. Thus satisfying relationships, sporting accomplishments, occupational or academic success and even the experience of warmth when cold, all promote DA release in the nucleus accumbens/ventral striatum and this is associated with the subjective experience of pleasure.

All drugs that are misused and that lead to dependence (with the notable exception of benzodiazepines) increase levels of DA in the nucleus accumbens. This criticality of DA in dependence is illustrated by:

- positron emission tomography research in humans which demonstrates that increased concentrations of DA in the brain mediate the pleasurable experiences associated with methylphenidate and cocaine (Volkow, 2004) and
- behavioural research in mice which demonstrates that DA D_2 receptor knockout mice self-administer alcohol to a lesser extent than wild type mice (Risinger et al, 2000).

Two further research findings are of note:

1. Whether an individual gains pleasure from drugs that are misused appears to depend on the concentration of DA D_2 receptors in the nucleus accumbens (Lingford-Hughes and Nutt, 2003). Individuals with low concentrations of DA D_2 receptors experience pleasure from such drugs, and may be predisposed to misuse them, while those with high concentrations do not.
2. It is not only the actual ingestion of alcohol or drugs that increases brain concentrations of DA. Even the mere anticipation of such ingestion will have this effect. This has led to the proposal that anticipated pleasure may depend upon DA D_2 receptors while actual experienced pleasure depends upon neurotransmitters including endorphins, gamma-amino butyric acid (GABA) and anandamide and upon opiate, GABA and cannabinoid receptors respectively (Burgdorf and Panksepp, 2005). If correct, this hypothesis has important implications for our understanding of alcohol and drug dependency.

It has long been hypothesised that DA D_3 receptors which are concentrated in the limbic system may be involved in the aetiology of alcohol, drug and nicotine misuse. However, it has not been possible to investigate this hypothesis because currently available DA receptor antagonists have affinity for both D_2 and D_3 receptors. Selective D_3 receptor antagonists have recently become available and their use in animal models of drug dependency suggest that DA D_3 receptors in the limbic system may play a significant role in drug dependency and that D_3 receptor antagonists may help in the treatment of drug-dependent people (Heidbreder et al, 2005).

A number of drugs that target the neurotransmitters or neuro-receptors discussed above have been developed in an attempt to treat alcohol, drug and nicotine misuse. The use of these and other drugs for this purpose will now be described and a number of drugs that are being developed will be commented upon.

The psychopharmacological treatment of alcohol, opiate and nicotine misuse

A growing number of drugs are available to help individuals withdraw from, and maintain abstinence from, alcohol, opiates and nicotine. These should be prescribed only as part of a programme of treatment that also includes education and counselling by members of a dedicated multidisciplinary team. There are as yet no clinical guidelines on the treatment of alcohol or drug misuse available from the National Institute for Clinical Excellence (NICE). Guidelines are available on the use of nicotine replacement therapy and bupropion for smoking cessation (see below) and guidelines are being developed on opiate detoxification.

Rapid and ultra-rapid opiate detoxification involving the administration of naltrexone while sedated or anaesthetised is not recommended by the UK Advisory Council on the Misuse of Drugs and will not be described in this volume.

Alcohol misuse

Psychotropic drugs have a place in the treatment of patients withdrawing from alcohol and in helping carefully selected patients maintain abstinence.

Alcohol withdrawal

Benzodiazepine drugs with a long duration of action will prevent or greatly diminish alcohol withdrawal symptoms. Chlordiazepoxide is widely used for this purpose (see Chapter 11). It is commonly prescribed at an initial dose of 40–200 mg daily in divided doses. This dose is then gradually reduced over 7–14 days. Chlormethiazole may be used in a similar manner to chlordiazepoxide but it is now only recommended for hospitalised patients.

Patients withdrawing from alcohol should be treated with thiamine or multivitamin preparations in addition to chlordiazepoxide or chlormethiazole. This is because alcohol-dependent individuals are frequently vitamin deficient and thiamine deficiency causes damage to the periaqueductal structures which leads to Wernicke's encephalopathy and Korsakoff's psychosis (see Wright and Sigmundsson, 2004).

Disulfiram

Disulfiram is approved as an adjuvant in the treatment of carefully selected and cooperative patients who misuse alcohol. Its absorption is variable and it is rapidly metabolised.

Disulfiram irreversibly inhibits acetaldehyde dehydrogenase, the enzyme responsible for the oxidation of acetaldehyde to acetate (Fig. 14.1). Disulfiram therefore causes acetaldehyde to accumulate in cells following ingestion of alcohol. This in turn causes facial flushing, severe headache, palpitations, tachycardia, hypertension, respiratory distress, nausea and vomiting. These symptoms commence within 15–30 minutes of ingesting alcohol and persist for several hours. Tachyarrhythmias, hypotension and collapse may occur if large quantities of alcohol are consumed and occasional deaths have been reported. The practice of 'alcohol challenge' in which the effects of disulfiram are demonstrated to a patient by administering a small quantity of alcohol is therefore strongly discouraged.

Patients must be alcohol free for at least 24 hours before disulfiram is administered and must remain alcohol free for at least 7 days after it is discontinued. Disulfiram is usually prescribed in an initial dose of 800 mg daily. This is gradually reduced over 5–7 days to a maintenance dose of 100–200 mg daily. Patients must be warned that a disulfiram/alcohol interaction may be triggered by the modest quantities of alcohol present in some foods, in cough remedies and in toiletries such as aftershave lotions. They should also be encouraged to carry a card advising that they are being treated with disulfiram.

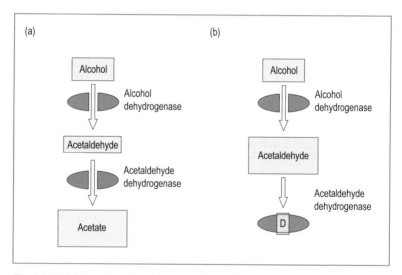

Fig. 14.1 (a) Alcohol is oxidised to acetaldehyde by alcohol dehydrogenase which in turn is oxidised to acetate by acetaldehyde dehydrogenase. (b) Disulfiram (D) irreversibly inhibits acetaldehyde dehydrogenase and causes acetaldehyde to accumulate and produce the typical disulfiram/alcohol interaction symptoms.

The adverse effects of disulfiram in the absence of alcohol include nausea, vomiting, drowsiness, halitosis, metallic taste and reduced libido. Dermatitis, hepatitis, peripheral neuritis and encephalopathy may also rarely occur. Disulfiram inhibits DA β hydroxylase, the enzyme responsible for the conversion of DA to noradrenaline (NA; norepinephrine). This effect elevates brain concentrations of DA and may both exacerbate schizophrenia and cause acute depressive, paranoid, schizophrenic or manic psychosis in otherwise healthy individuals.

Calcium carbide

The mechanism of action of calcium carbide is similar to that of disulfiram. It is no longer available in the UK.

Acamprosate

Acamprosate is approved in the UK for the maintenance of abstinence in patients who misuse alcohol. Its absorption is variable and it is neither bound to plasma proteins nor metabolised to any significant extent.

The chemical structure of acamprosate is similar to that of amino acids such as taurine and GABA. It must undergo acetylation before it can cross the blood–brain barrier. Its mechanism of action is thought to involve neuroinhibition via both an agonist effect at the GABA receptor and an antagonist effect at the glutamate receptor (Whitworth et al, 1996). It seems to reduce craving for alcohol and may help formerly dependent individuals maintain abstinence.

Treatment with acamprosate should be commenced as soon as possible after alcohol withdrawal. Once commenced, treatment should be continued for at least 1 year and should be maintained irrespective of further alcohol misuse during this year. Dosage depends on bodyweight. Individuals weighing more than 60 kg should take 666 mg three times daily (a cumulative daily dose of 1998 mg) while those weighing less than 60 kg should take 666 mg in the morning and 333 mg in the afternoon and evening (a cumulative daily dose of 1332 mg).

The adverse effects of acamprosate include nausea, vomiting, abdominal pain and diarrhoea. Itching, either with or without a maculopapular rash, may occur. Bullous skin disorders may rarely occur. Depression and alterations in libido have also been reported.

Naltrexone

Naltrexone (see below) is not approved in the UK for the treatment of alcohol misuse. It is approved for this indication in the US and is increasingly prescribed for it in the UK.

The mechanism of action of naltrexone in alcohol misuse is not understood but is presumed to involve opiate receptor blockade and thus neutralisation of the effects of endorphin release triggered by alcohol consumption.

Naltrexone is prescribed in a dosage of 50 mg daily for up to 12 weeks in the treatment of alcohol misuse. Naltrexone should only be prescribed for patients who have not taken opioids for at least 7–10 days (see below).

Opiate misuse

Methadone, buprenorphine and lofexidine are useful in withdrawing patients from opiates while naltrexone may help in maintaining abstinence following withdrawal.

Methadone

Methadone, in addition to its use as an analgesic, is also approved in the UK 'as a narcotic abstinence syndrome suppressant' in the treatment of opioid misuse. It is well absorbed from the gastrointestinal tract but undergoes extensive first pass metabolism. It reaches C_{MAX} in 4 hours and binds extensively to plasma proteins. Its $T_{1/2}$ is approximately 24 hours.

Methadone has high affinity for the μ opioid receptor at which it is an agonist. It has less marked affinity for the κ and δ opioid receptors at which it is also an agonist.

Clinically, methadone is a long-acting opioid agonist that may be substituted for diamorphine and that will prevent withdrawal symptoms. It is less sedating than morphine. It is usually administered orally but an injectable formulation is available. It should only be prescribed for individuals who are dependent upon opiates because it is intrinsically addictive. It is most often prescribed as an oral solution in a concentration of 1 mg per ml. The initial daily dose is 10–20 mg and this is increased by 10–20 mg per day until withdrawal symptoms have been controlled. The usual daily dose is then 40–60 mg which, given the long $T_{1/2}$, is administered once daily. Withdrawal is subsequently accomplished by gradually reducing the daily dosage at a rate that is agreed between the patient and the psychiatrist.

The adverse effects of methadone include nausea, vomiting, constipation and drowsiness. Sweating, arrhythmias, hypothermia, hallucinations, dysphoria and rash may also occur. Respiratory depression and hypotension only occur at relatively high doses or in combination with alcohol or other drugs. Methadone should not be administered with monoamine oxidase inhibitor antidepressant drugs or within 2 weeks of discontinuation of treatment with such drugs.

Buprenorphine

Buprenorphine is approved in the UK as 'substitution treatment for opioid drug dependence'. It is readily absorbed but is subject to extensive first pass metabolism. It must therefore be administered sublingually and it is important to instruct patients to allow buprenorphine tablets to be absorbed sublingually rather than swallowed. It reaches C_{MAX} in 2 hours and its $T_{1/2}$ is approximately 4 hours.

Buprenorphine is a partial agonist/antagonist at µ and, to a much lesser extent, κ opioid receptors. It will generally prevent withdrawal symptoms if substituted for diamorphine. However, it may precipitate withdrawal symptoms in patients dependent upon high doses of opiates because of its partial antagonist properties.

Buprenorphine is initially prescribed at a dose of 0.8–4.0 mg daily. This may be gradually increased to a maximum of 32 mg daily. Withdrawal from buprenorphine is subsequently accomplished by gradually reducing the daily dosage at a rate that is agreed between the patient and the psychiatrist. Buprenorphine may be prescribed in combination with methadone in which case it is recommended that the methadone dose be reduced to a maximum of 30 mg daily.

The adverse effects of buprenorphine are similar to those of methadone.

Lofexidine

Lofexidine is approved for 'the relief of symptoms in patients undergoing opiate detoxification'. It is readily absorbed and undergoes extensive hepatic metabolism. It reaches C_{MAX} in 3 hours and its $T_{1/2}$ is approximately 10 hours.

Lofexidine is an α_2 noradrenergic receptor agonist. It has high affinity for the α_{2A} receptor subtype and this may explain why it causes less hypotension than clonidine (see below). Lofexidine acts centrally to reduce NA secretion and thus reduce sympathetic tone. It will effectively prevent withdrawal symptoms in patients who are opiate dependent.

Lofexidine is usually prescribed in a dosage of 0.2 mg daily. This is gradually increased by 0.2–0.4 mg daily to a maximum dose of 2.4 mg daily. The usual duration of treatment is 7–10 days but longer periods of treatment are appropriate for some patients. Lofexidine should be discontinued gradually in order to prevent hypertensive episodes.

The adverse effects of lofexidine include dry mouth, throat and nose, drowsiness, bradycardia and hypotension (it should not be administered if the pulse rate is below 50 beats per minute and/or if systolic blood pressure is less than 90 mmHg). Sedation and coma may occur.

Clonidine

Clonidine is a non-selective α_2 noradrenergic receptor agonist that causes more hypotension than lofexidine (see above). It is occasionally used in a similar manner to lofexidine. However, it is not approved for this purpose in the UK and it is associated with a significant risk of severe hypotension and bradycardia.

Naltrexone

Naltrexone is approved as an 'adjunctive prophylactic therapy in the maintenance of detoxified, formerly opioid-dependent patients'. It is rapidly absorbed and undergoes extensive first pass metabolism. It reaches C_{MAX} in 1 hour and its $T_{1/2}$ is approximately 4 hours.

Naltrexone has both high specificity and high affinity for opioid receptors at which it is an antagonist. It neutralises the euphoriant effects of opiates when administered orally. It may therefore trigger withdrawal symptoms in opiate-dependent individuals. Naltrexone may help maintain abstinence in formerly opiate-dependent individuals. It may also be used for opiate withdrawal in hospitalised patients.

Naltrexone should only be prescribed for patients who have not taken opioids for at least 7–10 days. A naloxone challenge should be undertaken if recent opioid intake is suspected. Naloxone is a pure μ, κ and δ opioid receptor antagonist that will reverse the effect of opiates and cause an acute withdrawal syndrome, thus confirming recent opiate intake.

Naltrexone is prescribed at a dose of 25–50 mg daily. Once an appropriate daily dose has been determined the drug is usually administered on three days per week, a practice that is believed to improve compliance. Thus 100 mg on Monday and Wednesday and 150 mg on Friday may be prescribed. Treatment with naltrexone should be for 3 months in the first instance but some patients may require prolonged or even indefinite treatment.

The adverse effects of naltrexone include nausea, vomiting, anorexia, diarrhoea, abdominal pain, anxiety, headache, insomnia, fatigue, sweating, lacrimation, hypothermia, rash and sexual dysfunction.

Nicotine misuse

Individuals who wish to discontinue cigarette smoking may benefit from nicotine replacement therapy or bupropion. These should be prescribed in accordance with NICE guidelines (Box 14.1).

Nicotine replacement therapy

Several products are available that allow the administration of nicotine by sublingual (gum, lozenges), transdermal (patches) or transmucosal (nasal spray, inhaler) routes. The daily dosage of any product should be titrated to the quantity of cigarettes smoked daily, and may be maintained at this dosage for 3 months and then gradually reduced over a further period of 3 months.

Box 14.1: National Institute for Clinical Excellence guidelines on nicotine replacement therapy and bupropion for smoking cessation

nice guidelines

1. NICE has recommended (March 2002) that nicotine replacement therapy or bupropion should be prescribed only for a smoker who commits to a target stop date. The smoker should be offered advice and encouragement to aid smoking cessation.
2. Therapy to aid smoking cessation is chosen according to the smoker's likely compliance, availability of counselling and support, previous experience of smoking-cessation aids, contra-indications and adverse effects of the products, and the smoker's preferences.
3. Initial supply of the prescribed smoking-cessation therapy should be sufficient to last only 2 weeks after the target stop date; normally this will be 2 weeks of nicotine replacement therapy or 3–4 weeks of bupropion. A second prescription should be issued only if the smoker demonstrates a continuing attempt to stop smoking.
4. If an attempt to stop smoking is unsuccessful, the UK National Health Service should not normally fund a further attempt within 6 months.
5. There is currently insufficient evidence to recommend the combined use of nicotine replacement therapy and bupropion.

Nicotine products may cause nausea, hiccups, dyspepsia, headache, palpitations, insomnia, abnormal dreams, myalgia, anxiety and somnolence. Rash may occur with patches and ulceration of oropharyngeal mucosa has been reported.

Bupropion

Bupropion is approved 'as an aid to smoking cessation in combination with motivational support in nicotine-dependent patients'. It is approved for the treatment of depression in the US but not in the UK. It is rapidly absorbed and is metabolised to three active metabolites, hydroxybupropion, threohydrobupropion and erythrohydrobupropion. It reaches C_{MAX} in 3 hours, plasma protein binding is approximately 85% and its $T_{1/2}$ is approximately 20 hours. Bupropion is a pro-drug in that most of its effects are mediated by its metabolite, hydroxybupropion.

Bupropion is a NA and DA reuptake inhibitor. It does not inhibit the reuptake of serotonin and has no clinically significant effect at post-synaptic neuroreceptors. The mechanism of action of bupropion as an aid to smoking cessation is poorly understood but is probably mediated via NA and DA systems.

Bupropion should be commenced 2 weeks before an agreed smoking cessation date at an initial dose of 150 mg daily. The dose should be increased to 150 mg twice daily after 1 week and maintained

---

Box 14.2: Committee on Safety of Medicines advice on bupropion

The CSM has issued a reminder that bupropion is contra-indicated in patients with a history of seizures or of eating disorders, a CNS tumour, or who are experiencing acute symptoms of alcohol or benzodiazepine withdrawal. Bupropion should not be prescribed to patients with other risk factors for seizures unless the potential benefit of smoking cessation clearly outweighs the risk. Factors that increase the risk of seizures include concomitant administration of drugs that can lower the seizure threshold (e.g. antidepressants, antimalarials [such as mefloquine and chloroquine], antipsychotics, quinolones, sedating antihistamines, systemic corticosteroids, theophylline, tramadol), alcohol abuse, history of head trauma, diabetes, and use of stimulants and anorectics.

---

at this for a further 9 weeks. Bupropion should then be gradually discontinued.

The most common adverse effect associated with bupropion is insomnia. Others include gastrointestinal disturbance, impaired concentration, anxiety and alterations in taste. Rarely, psoriasis may be exacerbated and Stevens–Johnson syndrome and psychosis may occur. The Committee on Safety of Medicines (CSM) has advised that bupropion should not be administered to patients with a history of seizures or eating disorders (Box 14.2).

New treatments for alcohol, drug and nicotine misuse

Our advancing understanding of the psychopharmacology of alcohol, drug and nicotine misuse has led to the development of a number of new treatments for these disorders. Cannabinoid receptor antagonists utilise traditional drug technology while vaccines against cocaine and nicotine rely on novel science.

Cannabinoid receptor antagonists

Two cannabinoid neuroreceptors ($CB_{1 \& 2}$) and five endogenous cannabinoids or endocannabinoids have been identified (see Chapter 3). Rimonabant, a selective CB_1 receptor antagonist, has been investigated in obesity because cannabis smokers frequently experience intense hunger. It appears to be effective in the treatment of obesity and has also shown efficacy in smoking cessation. Other potential uses of CB_1 receptor antagonists include opiate and alcohol dependency.

Cocaine vaccines

Drugs that are misused must cross the blood–brain barrier and bind to receptors in the brain before they can exert their effects. A number of pharmaceutical and biotech companies are developing vaccines against cocaine in an attempt to find a permanent method of preventing it from crossing the blood–brain barrier. These vaccines consist of either:

- molecules that are antigenically identical to cocaine and that will induce an antibody response following injection or
- cocaine molecules bound to a carrier molecule in such a manner that an antibody response is induced following injection.

The antibodies generated by these vaccines bind specifically to cocaine and form antibody/cocaine complexes. The size of these complexes prevents them crossing the blood–brain barrier and cocaine is sequestered in the systemic circulation and excreted. Vaccinated individuals therefore do not experience any effect following administration of cocaine and the incentive to continue misusing cocaine is removed.

Nicotine vaccines

Nicotine vaccines with a similar mechanism of action to the cocaine vaccines described above are being developed. Cigarette smoking is legal in contrast to cocaine misuse, more individuals smoke cigarettes than misuse cocaine and, in contrast to cocaine, cigarette smoking causes several life-threatening diseases. The sociological and ethical questions raised by nicotine vaccines therefore differ profoundly from those raised by cocaine vaccines.

References and further reading

Burgdorf J, Panksepp J (2006) The neurobiology of positive emotions. Neuroscience and Biobehaviour Review 30(2):173–187.

Committee on Safety of Medicines (www.mca.gov.uk/aboutagency/regframework/csm/csmhome.htm) (accessed July 2005).

Heidbreder CA, Gardner EL, Xi ZX, Thanos PK, Mugnaini M, Hagan JJ, Ashby CR Jr (2005) The role of central dopamine D3 receptors in drug addiction: a review of pharmacological evidence. Brain Research Review 49(1):77–105.

Lingford-Hughes A, Nutt D (2003) Neurobiology of addiction and implications for treatment. British Journal of Psychiatry 182:97–100.

National Institute for Clinical Excellence (2002) Guidance on the use of nicotine replacement therapy (NRT) and bupropion for smoking cessation. (www.nice.org.uk) (accessed July 2005).

Risinger FO, Freeman PA, Rubinstein M, Low MJ, Grandy DK (2000) Lack of operant ethanol self-administration in dopamine D2 receptor knockout mice. Psychopharmacology 152(3):343–350.

Volkow N (2004) Drug dependence and addiction, III: Expectation and brain function in drug abuse. American Journal of Psychiatry 161(4):621.

Whitworth AB, Fischer F, Lesch OM, et al (1996) Comparison of acamprosate and placebo in long-term treatment of alcohol dependence. Lancet 25;347(9013):1438–1442.

Wright P, Sigmundsson T (2004) Organic psychiatry and epilepsy. In: Core Psychiatry (Eds Wright P, Phelan M and Stern J) (2nd Edition). London, Elsevier Saunders, pp. 381–411.

15

Parkinsonism and related disorders

Introduction

A significant proportion of patients treated with typical antipsychotic (AP) drugs, a significantly smaller proportion treated with atypical AP drugs, and some patients treated with tricyclic and selective serotonin reuptake inhibiting antidepressant drugs or with lithium, develop acute dystonia, Parkinsonism, akathisia or tardive dyskinesia (see Chapter 8).

These extrapyramidal system (EPS) adverse effects cause personal distress and functional disability, and militate against future compliance with prophylactic AP treatment thereby increasing patients' risk of relapse. EPS adverse effects are also stigmatising – patients suffering with them look and behave abnormally and this impacts upon social acceptance and rehabilitation. It is probable therefore that the single most important advantage of atypical over typical AP drugs is their greatly reduced propensity for causing EPS adverse effects.

Parkinson's disease is caused by a deficiency of DA and a relative excess of cholinergic neurotransmission at muscarinic neuroreceptors in the basal ganglia. It has been treated with synthetic derivatives of belladonna alkaloids that inhibit cholinergic muscarinic neurotransmission in a similar manner to atropine for almost 80 years. These drugs have almost no activity at the nicotinic receptor. Drugs that enhance dopaminergic neurotransmission in the basal ganglia are a more recent development. These may exacerbate psychotic symptoms and are not effective in alleviating the EPS adverse effects associated with AP drugs so they will not be discussed further.

Table 15.1: The daily dose range and available formulations of the anticholinergic (antimuscarinic) drugs approved in the UK

Drug	Dose range	Available formulations
Benzatropine	0.5–6 mg orally, 1–2 mg intramuscular or intravenous	Tablets Injection
Benzhexol (trihexyphenidyl hydrochloride)	1–15 mg	Tablets Liquid
Orphenadrine	150–400 mg	Tablets Liquid
Procyclidine	7.5–30 mg	Tablets Liquid Injection

Anticholinergic drugs

The anticholinergic (or more correctly antimuscarinic) drugs approved in the UK include benzatropine, benzhexol (or trihexyphenidyl hydrochloride), orphenadrine and procyclidine (see Table 15.1). Biperiden is no longer available.

Pharmacokinetics

In general, anticholinergic drugs are well absorbed from the gastrointestinal tract. They are metabolised in the liver. Most have a T_{MAX} of 1–2 hours and a $T_{1/2}$ of approximately 12 hours.

Procyclidine is slowly absorbed from the gastrointestinal tract (and should be administered by intramuscular or intravenous injection in an emergency) and has a T_{MAX} of 6–8 hours. Benzatropine has a longer duration of action and a cumulative effect when compared with other anticholinergic drugs. Orphenadrine has a $T_{1/2}$ of up to 20 hours (see below).

Pharmacodynamics

Dopamine (DA)-secreting neurones extend in the nigrostriatal tract from the substantia nigra to the striatum (Fig. 15.1). In the striatum, these DA neurones synapse with acetylcholine (Ach)-secreting neurones that have their cell bodies in the caudate and putamen. These Ach neurones ultimately project to the premotor cortex thereby

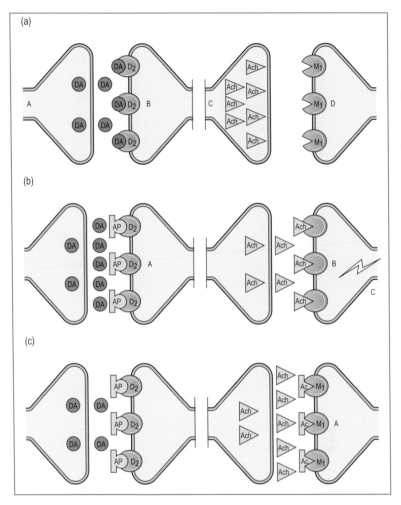

Fig. 15.1 Physiological role of dopamine and acetylcholine in the striatum and the mechanism of action of antipsychotic drugs in causing, and of anticholinergic drugs in alleviating, dystonia and Parkinsonism. (**a**) Dopaminergic fibres from the substantia nigra (A) release dopamine (DA) which binds to DA D_2 receptors on the cell bodies of striatal cholinergic neurones (B). This inhibits the cholinergic neurones from releasing acetylcholine (Ach) into the synapse (C) and prevents activation of postsynaptic muscarinic M_1 receptors (D). Thus the physiological role of DA in the striatum is to suppress cholinergic activity. (**b**) Antipsychotic drugs (AP) block DA D_2 receptors on the cell bodies of striatal cholinergic neurones, preventing their inhibition by DA (A). Ach is released and binds to postsynaptic muscarinic M_1 receptors (B). Depolarisation of postsynaptic neurones (C) is associated with dystonia and Parkinsonism. (**c**) Anticholinergic drugs block muscarinic M_1 receptors (A) and prevent Ach from activating the postsynaptic neurone. This effect is associated with alleviation of dystonia and Parkinsonism.

permitting the striatum to monitor and modulate voluntary movements. The activity of these Ach neurones is inhibited by DA from nigrostriatal fibres binding to DA D_2 receptors on their cell bodies. This inhibition is prevented by DA D_2 receptor antagonists such as AP drugs. This causes a relative excess of Ach neurotransmission at muscarinic M_1 neuroreceptors and this in turn may lead to acute dystonia and Parkinsonism.

Anticholinergic drugs both prevent and alleviate EPS adverse effects caused by excess Ach neurotransmission by blocking muscarinic M_1 neuroreceptors. Biperiden and procyclidine are the most selective of the anticholinergic drugs for M_1 neuroreceptors and benzhexol the least selective.

The atypical AP drugs are much less likely to cause EPS adverse effects than the typical AP drugs and even within the typical and atypical classes of AP drugs, some drugs are less likely to cause EPS adverse effects than others. These differences in EPS liability may be accounted for by anticholinergic activity and/or serotonin $5HT_{2A}$ receptor antagonism that is an intrinsic property of individual AP drugs.

Intrinsic anticholinergic activity

Most typical and some atypical AP drugs block muscarinic M_1 neuroreceptors. While this action causes troublesome adverse effects such as dry mouth and blurred vision, it also serves to alleviate EPS adverse effects by reducing the effect of excess Ach neurotransmission (see above).

Intrinsic serotonin $5HT_{2A}$ receptor antagonism

Most atypical and some typical AP drugs have relatively high affinity for $5HT_{2A}$ receptors on the cell bodies and terminal axon fibres of DA-secreting neurones in the basal ganglia (see Chapter 8). Occupancy of these receptors by 5HT inhibits the release of DA while their blockade by AP drugs with intrinsic serotonin $5HT_{2A}$ receptor antagonism prevents 5HT from exerting its inhibitory effect and increases dopaminergic activity in the basal ganglia (see Fig. 8.3).

Efficacy

Anticholinergic drugs are not required by the majority of patients treated with atypical AP drugs. They should not be prescribed prophylactically for patients taking typical AP drugs because:

- while a significant proportion of such individuals will develop EPS adverse effects, not all will
- anticholinergic drugs impair the therapeutic effect of AP drugs

- anticholinergic drugs may cause psychosis, confusion (especially in high dosage and/or in elderly patients) and acute organic reaction
- anticholinergic drugs have euphoriant and stimulant properties and may cause dependence and
- anticholinergic drugs may increase the risk of developing tardive dyskinesia.

The syndromes of acute dystonia, Parkinsonism, akathisia and tardive dyskinesia are described in Chapter 8. Their treatment is now described.

Acute dystonia and Parkinsonism

Anticholinergic drugs are rapidly effective in acute dystonia and may be administered by intramuscular or intravenous injection (benzatropine and procyclidine) if a more rapid effect is desired or if swallowing is difficult because of oropharyngeal muscle spasm. Once acute dystonia has been successfully treated, consideration should be given to either reducing the dose of AP drug or switching a patient being treated with a typical AP drug to an atypical AP drug. Prophylactic anticholinergic medication should only be prescribed if these changes are not effective or not possible.

Anticholinergic drugs gradually reduce the symptoms of Parkinsonism. Once Parkinsonism has been successfully treated, consideration should be given to reducing the dose of AP drug or switching a patient being treated with a typical AP drug to an atypical AP drug. Prophylactic anticholinergic medication should only be prescribed if these changes are not effective or not possible.

The anticholinergic drugs appear to be equally effective in alleviating acute dystonia and Parkinsonism. Therefore when treatment with an anticholinergic drug is required, the choice of drug should be based on both the method of administration that is necessary (only benzatropine and procyclidine are available in injectable formulations) and safety and tolerability considerations.

Akathisia

Akathisia occurs in up to 50% of patients treated with typical AP drugs. It responds variably to anticholinergic drugs and the most appropriate management strategies are either reducing the dose of AP drug or switching a patient being treated with a typical AP drug to an atypical AP drug. If these changes are not effective or not possible treatment with beta-blocking medication or benzodiazepines may be considered.

It is very important to diagnose and treat akathisia because it is extremely distressing to patients, both physically and psychologically, because it militates against future compliance with prophylactic AP drug treatment and thereby increasing patients' risk of relapse and because it is potentially associated with an increased risk of suicide (Hansen, 2001).

Tardive dyskinesia

There are no satisfactory treatments for tardive dyskinesia. Anticholinergic drugs should be avoided because they are not effective and probably worsen it (this is also why they should not be prescribed prophylactically for every patient treated with AP drugs). Prevention is therefore critically important and is best achieved by use of atypical AP drugs. Treatment strategies in patients with established tardive dyskinesia include:

- very slowly reducing the dose of AP drug
- switching patients being treated with typical AP drugs to atypical AP drugs. The risk of tardive dyskinesia is considerably less with atypical AP drugs compared with typical AP drugs. For example one double blind study reported that 0.5% of 513 olanzapine-treated and 7.5% of 114 haloperidol-treated patients developed tardive dyskinesia during 1 year of observation (Beasley et al, 1999)
- switching patients being treated with typical or atypical AP drugs to clozapine. It should be noted that clozapine is approved in the UK for the treatment of patients with schizophrenia 'who have severe, untreatable neurological adverse reactions to other antipsychotic agents, including atypical antipsychotics'.

Safety

The adverse effects of anticholinergic drugs include nausea, constipation, drowsiness, dry mouth, blurred vision, dilated pupils, confusion and hallucinations. Narrow angle glaucoma may worsen and acute urinary retention may occur in patients with prostatic hypertrophy.

Orphenadrine has marked membrane-stabilising effects and a $T_{1/2}$ of up to 20 hours. These factors combine to generate a lethal dose which may be no more than 10 times the therapeutic dose. It therefore probably has no place in psychiatric practice and should certainly be avoided in patients at risk of overdosing or suicide.

Anticholinergic drugs have a stimulant effect and may cause euphoria. They are therefore widely abused both by patients for whom they are prescribed and by other individuals. This euphoriant effect is most evident with benzhexol and procyclidine. Indeed it has become increasingly evident that benzhexol is widely used by suicide bombers to induce a sense of euphoria and invulnerability both during their training and when engaged in their final actions (Ridolfo, 2004).

Sudden discontinuation of treatment with anticholinergic drugs can cause cholinergic rebound characterised by restlessness, insomnia, diarrhoea, abdominal pain, movement disorder and salivation. Anticholinergic drugs should therefore be gradually discontinued.

References and further reading

Beasley CM, Dellva MA, Tamura RN, Morgenstern H, Glazer WM, Ferguson K, Tollefson GD (1999) Randomised double-blind comparison of the incidence of tardive dyskinesia in patients with schizophrenia during long-term treatment with olanzapine or haloperidol. British Journal of Psychiatry 174:23–30.

Hansen L (2001) A critical review of akathisia, and its possible association with suicidal behaviour. Human Psychopharmacology 16(7):495–505.

Ridolfo K (2004) Radio Free Europe Inside Iraq. Volume 7, number 11. Available online at www.rferl.org/reports/iraq-report/2004/03/11-260304.asp (accessed July 2005).

16

Alzheimer's disease and other dementias

Introduction

Four drugs are currently approved in the UK for the symptomatic treatment of Alzheimer's dementia. Three of these are acetyl-cholinesterase inhibitors while one is an N-methyl, D-aspartate (NMDA) receptor antagonist. A number of other drugs that are not specifically approved for this purpose are also occasionally used and should be regarded as investigational drugs at this time. In addition, several drugs are used to prevent and treat vascular dementia.

The psychopharmacology of Alzheimer's disease

Alzheimer's disease is characterised by senile plaques and neuro-fibrillary tangles accompanied by loss of neurones in the frontal and temporal cortex. It is important for the psychiatrist to realize that Alzheimer's disease is not an 'acetylcholine (Ach) disorder' but rather a disease that causes a generalised loss of all neurones and of all neuro-transmitters throughout the brain. Nonetheless, the most obvious neuronal loss in Alzheimer's disease is of cholinergic neurones in the nucleus of Meynert, the largest cholinergic nucleus, and in other basal nuclei. These neuropathological changes are associated with reduced activity of choline acetyltransferase, the enzyme that catalyses the conversion of choline and acetyl-CoA to Ach (Figs 16.1 and 16.2). This leads to reduced Ach production which in turn correlates with cognitive impairment.

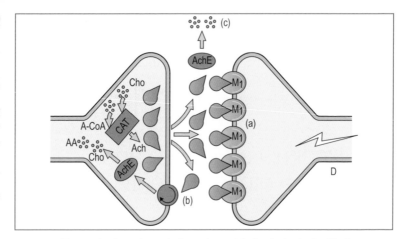

Fig. 16.1 The synthesis and metabolism of acetylcholine in the brain. Choline acetyltransferase (CAT) catalyses the conversion of choline (Cho) and acetyl-CoA (A-CoA) to acetylcholine (Ach) which is released into the synapse. Ach then either (**a**) binds to post-synaptic muscarinic receptors (predominantly M_1) causing the neurone to depolarise (D), (**b**) binds to the Ach reuptake transporter protein on the presynaptic membrane via which it enters the terminal axon fibre and is catabolised to acetic acid (AA) and Cho by acetylcholinesterase (AchE) or (**c**) is catabolised by AchE in the synapse.

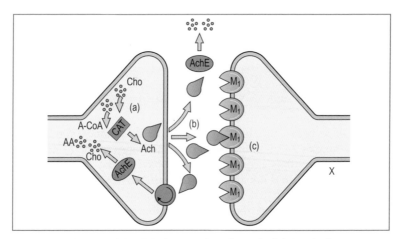

Fig. 16.2 Reduced activity of choline acetyltransferase in Alzheimer's disease. Neuronal loss in the nucleus of Meynert and other basal nuclei in patients with Alzheimer's disease is associated with reduced activity of CAT (indicated by the diminished rectangle) (**a**). This causes a reduction in Ach synthesis and a reduced concentration of Ach in the synapse (**b**) and at the postsynaptic muscarinic M_1 receptors (**c**). Consequently, the neurone does not depolarise (X).

Acetylcholinesterase is present in both the terminal axon fibres of cholinergic neurones and in the synapse. It catalyses the metabolism of Ach to acetic acid and choline (Fig. 16.1). Acetylcholinesterase inhibitors were therefore developed in the hope that their use would increase Ach levels in the brain by inhibition of its degradative enzyme and would thereby reduce the symptoms of Alzheimer's disease (Fig. 16.3). The first such drug to be developed, the tetrahydro-aminoacridine tacrine, was found to be effective and was approved in the UK. However, it subsequently proved to be hepatotoxic and was withdrawn from use. It remains available in the US. Donepezil, rivastigmine and galantamine are the three acetylcholinesterase inhibitors that are currently approved for use in the UK.

Concentrations of the excitatory amino acid, glutamate, and of its NMDA neuroreceptors are increased in Alzheimer's disease. This causes abnormal glutamatergic neurotransmission at NMDA neuro-receptors which both contributes to the symptoms of Alzheimer's disease and promotes disease progression because excess glutamate is neurotoxic. NMDA receptor antagonists have been developed in the hope that their use would both reduce patients' symptoms and block the neurotoxic effects of excess glutamate. Memantine is the only NMDA receptor antagonist that is currently approved for use in the UK.

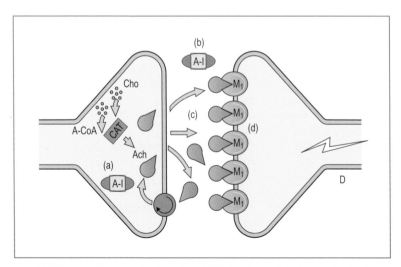

Fig. 16.3 The mechanism of action of acetylcholinesterase inhibitors in the treatment of Alzheimer's disease. AchE inhibitors (AI) reduce the activity of AchE in both the terminal axon fibres (**a**) and in the synapse (**b**). This reduces the rate of catabolism of Ach, increasing its concentration in the synapse (**c**) and at postsynaptic M_1 receptors (**d**), and permitting depolarisation of the neurone (D).

The synthesis of serotonin (5HT), dopamine (DA) and noradrenaline (NA; norepinephrine) and of the inhibitory amino acid gamma-aminobutyric acid (GABA) is reduced in Alzheimer's disease as are numbers of 5HT (particularly $5HT_2$) neuroreceptors. Drugs designed to reverse these neurotransmitter and neuroreceptor changes are under development but none is yet approved for clinical use.

Acetylcholinesterase inhibitors

Donepezil, galantamine and rivastigmine have a similar mechanism of action and similar efficacy and safety profiles. The efficacy of these acetylcholinesterase inhibitors in the symptomatic treatment of Alzheimer's dementia will now be discussed. This will be followed by a commentary on each of the three drugs in turn.

Efficacy of acetylcholinesterase inhibitors

A significant number of clinical trials have investigated the efficacy of acetylcholinesterase inhibitors in patients with Alzheimer's disease. In general, these demonstrate that both cognitive and functional impairment are either improved or stabilised in approximately 50% of patients with mild to moderately severe Alzheimer's dementia as measured by a Mini Mental-State Examination (MMSE) score of ≥ 12.

It is believed that this improvement/stabilisation is caused by increased synaptic concentrations of Ach consequent upon inhibition of acetylcholinesterase. Delaying the metabolism of Ach can therefore compensate for the reduced production of Ach that is characteristic of Alzheimer's disease. With disease progression, however, Ach synthesis decreases to a level beyond which inhibition of acetylcholinesterase can no longer compensate. This is accompanied by progression of cognitive and functional impairment.

Treatment with acetylcholinesterase inhibitors should only be initiated by a specialist experienced in the diagnosis and treatment of patients with dementia. Cognitive assessments should be undertaken before treatment commences and approximately 3 months later. Treatment should then be discontinued if cognitive impairment has not either improved or stabilised. It is usual to undertake a further cognitive assessment 1–2 months after discontinuing treatment and to consider recommencing treatment if significant deterioration has occurred during that period. Patients who respond to acetylcholinesterase inhibitors should continue to take them while their MMSE score, evaluated approximately every 6 months, remains ≥ 12.

The National Institute for Clinical Excellence (NICE), based on the results of 13 clinical trials (5 each for donepezil and rivastigmine and

3 for galantamine), recommended the use of acetylcholinesterase inhibitors for the symptomatic treatment of mild to moderate Alzheimer's disease in 2001 (Box 16.1). Following a further review, NICE made a preliminary recommendation that neither acetylcholinesterase inhibitors nor memantine are appropriate treatments for Alzheimer's disease (NICE, 2005a). The Faculty of Old Age Psychiatry of the Royal College of Psychiatrists (2005) expressed 'severe disappointment' with this preliminary recommendation. In January 2006 NICE made a further preliminary recommendation that acetylcholinesterase inhibitors but not memantine should be considered in the treatment of Alzheimer's disease of moderate severity (MMSE 10–20) (NICE 2006). Readers should note, however, that the 2001 NICE recommendations remain in force until final updated guidance is issued.

The efficacy of the NMDA receptor antagonist, memantine, is discussed below. Its use is being evaluated by NICE as part of the review of treatment for Alzheimer's disease referred to above.

---

nice guidelines

Box 16.1: National Institute of Clinical Excellence guidance on the use of acetylcholinesterase inhibitors in Alzheimer's disease (2001)

NICE has recommended that, for the adjunctive treatment of mild and moderate Alzheimer's disease in those whose Mini Mental-State Examination (MMSE) score is above 12 points, donepezil, galantamine and rivastigmine should be available under the following conditions:

1. Alzheimer's disease must be diagnosed in a specialist clinic; the clinic should also assess cognitive, global and behavioural functioning, activities of daily living, and the likelihood of compliance with treatment.
2. Treatment should be initiated by specialists but may be continued by general practitioners under a shared-care protocol.
3. The carers' views of the condition should be sought before and during drug treatment.
4. The patient should be assessed 2–4 months after a maintenance dose is established; drug treatment should continue only if the MMSE score has improved or has not deteriorated *and* if behavioural or functional assessment shows improvement.
5. The patient should be assessed every 6 months and drug treatment should normally continue only if the MMSE score remains above 12 points and if treatment is considered to have a worthwhile effect on the global, functional and behavioural condition.

Donepezil

Donepezil is approved for the symptomatic treatment of mild to moderately severe Alzheimer's dementia.

Pharmacokinetics

Donepezil is almost completely absorbed in the upper gastrointestinal tract. It has a T_{MAX} of 3 hours. It is metabolised by cytochrome P450 enzymes with production of the active metabolite, 6-O-desmethyldonepezil. Plasma protein binding is approximately 95% and its $T_{1/2}$ is 3 days.

Donepezil is only available as tablets. It should be administered in a dose of 5–10 mg once daily.

Pharmacodynamics

Donepezil, a piperidine, is a specific, non-competitive and reversible inhibitor of acetylcholinesterase. Donepezil has been demonstrated to inhibit the activity of acetylcholinesterase in red blood cells by approximately 70% and it is assumed that similar inhibition occurs in the brain. Inhibition of red cell acetylcholinesterase correlates with improvements in cognition. Donepezil inhibits acetylcholinesterase one thousand times more potently than peripheral Ach-degrading enzymes such as butyrycholinesterase.

Safety

Donepezil may cause gastrointestinal (nausea, vomiting, anorexia, diarrhoea) and central nervous system (fatigue, headache, insomnia, dizziness, convulsions, neuroleptic malignant syndrome and depression) adverse effects. It may also cause rash.

The cholinomimetic effects of acetylcholinesterase inhibitors like donepezil may exacerbate (or induce *de novo*):

- urinary retention
- syncope, bradycardia and atrioventricular block (this effect may potentiate the effects of drugs that reduce pulse rate such as digoxin)
- seizures and
- may cause a worsening of Parkinson's disease and other extrapyramidal disorders including drug-induced Parkinsonism.

Galantamine

Like donepezil, galantamine is approved for the symptomatic treatment of mild to moderately severe Alzheimer's dementia.

Pharmacokinetics

Galantamine is rapidly absorbed and has a T_{MAX} of 2 hours. It is metabolised in the liver and plasma protein binding is approximately 20%. Its $T_{1/2}$ is 7 hours.

Galantamine is available in tablet and liquid formulations. It should be administered in a dose of 8–12 mg twice daily.

Pharmacodynamics

Galantamine is a reversible competitive inhibitor of acetylcholinesterase with a similar mechanism of action to donepezil. The maximum inhibition of acetylcholinesterase activity achieved with galantamine is approximately 40%. Unlike donepezil, galantamine is also a nicotinic neuroreceptor agonist.

Safety

Galantamine has a similar adverse effects profile to donepezil.

Rivastigmine

Like donepezil and galantamine, rivastigmine is approved for the symptomatic treatment of mild to moderately severe Alzheimer's dementia.

Pharmacokinetics

Rivastigmine is rapidly and completely absorbed and has a T_{MAX} of 1 hour. It is metabolised in the liver and plasma protein binding is approximately 40%. Its $T_{1/2}$ is 1.5 hours.

Rivastigmine is available in capsule and liquid formulations. It should be administered in a dose of 3–6 mg twice daily.

Pharmacodynamics

Rivastigmine is a pseudo-irreversible non-competitive inhibitor of acetylcholinesterase with a similar mechanism of action to donepezil. The maximum inhibition of acetylcholinesterase activity achieved with rivastigmine is approximately 60%.

Safety

Rivastigmine has a similar adverse effects profile to donepezil.

N-methyl D-aspartate receptor antagonists

Memantine is the only NMDA receptor antagonist approved in the UK for the symptomatic treatment of dementia in Alzheimer's disease.

N-methyl D-aspartate receptor antagonists

Memantine

In contrast to the acetylcholinesterase inhibitors which are approved for the symptomatic treatment of mild to moderately severe Alzheimer's dementia, memantine is approved in the UK for the symptomatic treatment of moderately severe to severe Alzheimer's dementia.

Pharmacokinetics

Memantine is completely absorbed in the upper gastrointestinal tract. It has a T_{MAX} of 3–8 hours. Plasma protein binding is approximately 45% and its $T_{1/2}$ is 3–5 days.

Memantine is available in tablets and liquid formulations. It should be administered in a dose of 10 mg twice daily.

Pharmacodynamics

It is believed that prolonged activation of NMDA receptors by the excitatory amino acid, glutamate, is responsible for both some of the symptoms of Alzheimer's dementia and, perhaps more importantly, for disease progression. Memantine is a non-competitive NMDA receptor antagonist that binds preferentially to NMDA receptor gated ionotropic (cation) channels. This action is thought to inhibit the neurotoxic effects of excess glutamate. Memantine is also an antagonist at both $5HT_3$ and at nicotinic neuroreceptors.

Efficacy

The clinical trials undertaken with memantine have evaluated its effect on cognition (using the Alzheimer's Disease Cooperative Study Activities of Daily Living inventory or ADCS ADL) and daily functioning (using the Severe Impairment Battery or SIB) in patients with moderately severe to severe Alzheimer's dementia as measured by a MMSE score ≤14.

One randomised, double-blind trial involved 252 patients (66% female) with a mean age of 76 years who were treated with memantine 20 mg daily or placebo for 28 weeks. Memantine was superior to placebo on both the ADCS ADL and the SIB and also on a clinician-rated measure of change, the Clinicians Interview-Based Impression of Change. These results indicate that memantine is associated with either improvement in, or a slower deterioration in, cognition and daily functioning. A total of 29% and 10% of patients in this trial were deemed to have responded to memantine and placebo respectively.

A second randomised, double-blind trial involved 404 patients (66% female) with a mean age of 76 years who had already been treated for at least 6 months with donepezil. Treatment with donepezil was continued and they were additionally treated with memantine 20 mg daily or placebo for 24 weeks. Memantine with donepezil was superior to placebo with donepezil on the ADCS ADL.

A recent review of double-blind, placebo-controlled, randomized clinical trials of memantine in patients with moderate to severe Alzheimer's dementia concluded that a small beneficial effect on cognition, activities of daily living and behaviour was present after six months (Areosa et al, 2005).

Safety

The common adverse effects of memantine include headache, dizziness, confusion and hallucinations. Anxiety, vomiting, cystitis and seizures have also been reported.

Concomitant administration of memantine and amantadine should be avoided because of the risk of psychosis. Memantine does not affect the inhibition of acetylcholinesterase by donepezil, galantamine or rivastigmine.

Investigational drugs for the treatment of dementia

These include a number of drugs that are occasionally used as follows:

- Anti-inflammatory (based on Schneider's 1996 report that Alzheimer's disease is less common in patients with rheumatoid arthritis) and antioxidant drugs.
- Oestrogens.
- Neuroprotective drugs or nootropics such as piracetam (more frequently used to treat cortical myoclonus) and co-dergocrine (a cerebral vasodilator licensed as an adjunctive treatment in mild to moderate dementia).

A number of drugs are also in development including:

- Neuroprotective drugs that modify glutamate transmission.
- Agents that modify the deposition of amyloid and tau protein in plaques and neurofibrillary tangles.
- Antibodies directed at plaques and neurofibrillary tangles.

Gene therapy for Alzheimer's disease in which the gene for nerve growth factor (contained within a viral vector) is injected directly into the nucleus basalis of Meynert is currently being investigated.

Vascular dementia

Cerebrovascular disease can both exacerbate Alzheimer's disease and cause a discrete vascular dementia in the absence of other pathology.

Measures aimed at preventing cerebrovascular disease (or at preventing its progression if it is already evident) will therefore prevent (or prevent the progression of) vascular dementia. Such measures include:

- Cessation of cigarette smoking.
- Management of obesity.
- Prophylactic use of drugs that reduce platelet adhesiveness (aspirin, dipyridamole).
- Identification and treatment of hypertension, diabetes mellitus and hyperlipidaemia.

A review of vascular dementia and its treatment is provided by Shah and Tovey (2005).

References and further reading

Areosa SA, Sherriff F, McShane R (2005) Memantine for dementia. Cochrane Database Systematic Review 20(3):CD003154.

National Institute for Clinical Excellence (2001) Donepezil, rivastigmine and galantamine for the treatment of Alzheimer's disease. Online. Available at: www.nice.org.uk (accessed July 2005).

National Institute for Clinical Excellence (2005a) Appraisal Consultation Document. Donepezil, rivastigmine, galantamine and memantine for the treatment of Alzheimer's disease. Available at: www.nice.org.uk (accessed July 2005).

National Institute for Clinical Excellence (2005b) Update on Alzheimer's appraisal. Online. Available at: www.nice.org.uk (accessed July 2005).

National Institute for Clinical Excellence (2006) NICE consults on revised first draft guidance on the use of drugs to treat Alzheimer's disease (press release). Available at: www.nice.org.uk/pdf/2006_001_Alz_Press_rellease_AD–App_Jan_06.pdf

Royal College of Psychiatrists (2005)

Schneider LS (1996) New therapeutic approaches to Alzheimer's disease. Journal of Clinical Psychiatry 57(Suppl 14):30–36.

Shah A, Tovey E (2005) Psychiatry of old age. In: Core Psychiatry (2nd Edition) (Eds Wright P, Stern J, Phelan M). London: Saunders, pp. 481–492.

17

Electroconvulsive therapy, phototherapy and transcranial magnetic stimulation

Introduction

In addition to drugs, three further physical treatments are utilised in the battle against psychiatric illness. These are electroconvulsive therapy (ECT), phototherapy and transcranial magnetic stimulation (TMS). ECT is the most extensively utilised of these treatments while TMS must currently be regarded as an experimental treatment.

A discussion of neurosurgery which is occasionally employed in the treatment of psychiatric disorders is beyond the scope of this volume but Cooney (2005) provides an excellent review.

Electroconvulsive therapy

ECT, the passing of a brief electrical stimulus through the brain under carefully controlled conditions in order to induce a generalised seizure for therapeutic purposes, is probably the most controversial treatment prescribed by psychiatrists. Yet it is probably the most effective and safest treatment available for depressed patients and it may be life saving.

Mechanism of action of electroconvulsive therapy

The mechanism of action of ECT is unknown. Early hypotheses drew upon psychodynamic theory and suggested that the amnesia induced by ECT erased the traumatic memories responsible for depression. More recent hypotheses have focused on the effect of generalised seizures on neurophysiology, neurochemistry and neuroendocrinology.

Electroconvulsive therapy and neurophysiology

The electroencephalogram (EEG) during an application of ECT is similar to that recorded during a generalised seizure with spike phenomena and slow (δ and θ) waves which are soon followed by flattening of the EEG. These changes are most evident over the dominant hemisphere and they persist for an increasingly longer duration after subsequent applications of ECT. Very high-voltage slow waves appear towards the end of a course of ECT and the α rhythm may disappear. These changes may persist for up to 3 months following a course of ECT but while they are well documented, they are not well understood.

ECT has an anticonvulsant action in that subsequent applications increase the seizure threshold. The kindling theory of mood disorder states that episodes of illness are caused by seizure-inducing electrical activity in the brain which occurs following previous episodes of subthreshold electrical activity. This and the fact that several anti-epileptic drugs are effective treatments for mood disorder has led to the suggestion that ECT may exert its beneficial effect via its anticonvulsant properties. On the other hand antidepressant (AD) drugs do not raise the seizure threshold and benzodiazepine drugs, while effective in treating epilepsy, are ineffective in treating depression.

So while seizures are necessary if ECT is to have a beneficial effect, they are not sufficient. An electrical stimulus that just exceeds the seizure threshold will induce a seizure but will not alleviate depression and in fact an effective stimulus must exceed the seizure threshold by 100–200% (see below). Thus it may be that the electrical stimulus exerts its therapeutic effect via the non-seizure mechanisms outlined below and that seizures are epiphenomena. Indeed the electrical stimulus itself is not essential and seizures induced by drugs such as metrazol are also effective (see Chapter 2).

Electroconvulsive therapy and neurochemistry

The serotonergic (5HT), noradrenergic (NA) and dopaminergic (DA) hypotheses of depression have been discussed in Chapter 9. In general, it is accepted that ECT alters the responsivity of postsynaptic neuroreceptors to neurotransmitters. Specifically, ECT:

- causes downregulation of postsynaptic $5HT_2$ neuroreceptors, an effect it shares with AD drugs, and sensitisation of presynaptic $5HT_{1A\,\&\,3}$ receptors. ECT also increases levels of the 5HT metabolite, HIAA, in cerebrospinal fluid
- causes downregulation of NA β receptors and induces a transient increase in plasma NA and
- increases levels of the DA metabolite, HVA, in cerebrospinal fluid.

So while ECT causes some neurochemical changes that are similar to those caused by AD drugs, ECT has other effects that differ significantly from those of such drugs. It will be apparent from this brief overview that our understanding of the neurochemical changes induced by ECT is limited.

Electroconvulsive therapy and neuroendocrinology

Neuroendocrine abnormalities are common in depression and hypercortisolaemia in particular has been implicated in the weight loss, sleep disturbance, loss of libido and cognitive impairment many depressed patients experience.

As noted above, it may be that the seizures induced by ECT are not directly involved in its efficacy and it has been hypothesised that the electrical stimulus administered has a direct effect on the hypothalamus that causes a surge in the secretion of hormones. For example prolactin secretion is well known to increase following ECT (as well as following generalised epileptic seizures). This hormonal surge appears to normalise the hypothalamo–pituitary–adrenal axis which in turn restores appetite, sleep, libido and cognition to normal.

Efficacy

Indications for electroconvulsive therapy

ECT is primarily indicated for the treatment of depression. It is also occasionally employed in the treatment of catatonic schizophrenia and mania. Indeed there was no effective treatment for mania before the advent of ECT, other than the passage of time.

The National Institute for Clinical Excellence (NICE) (2003) recommends ECT for severe depressive illness, catatonia (both in schizophrenia and in depression) and a prolonged or severe manic episode. With the exception of catatonia, NICE does not recommend ECT for the general management of schizophrenia. NICE further recommends that ECT is used only to achieve rapid and short-term improvement of severe symptoms after:

- an adequate trial of other treatment options has proven ineffective and/or
- when the condition is considered to be potentially life-threatening.

What constitutes 'an adequate trial of other treatment' for depression? Treatment-resistant depression is discussed in Chapter 9 where it is noted that ECT would generally be considered before triple AD drug therapy or the addition of thyroxine to an AD drug. It is further noted that most psychiatrists would consider ECT if treatment with two different newer AD drugs prescribed in adequate doses for an adequate duration of time proved ineffective.

Ensuring the effectiveness of electroconvulsive therapy

The administration and monitoring of ECT is fully described by Freeman (1995) and a review is provided by Cooney (2005). If it is to be effective ECT must induce a seizure which is generalised (as evidenced by bilateral clonic limb movements) and of sufficient duration ($\geq$15 seconds of visible bilateral clonic limb movements or $\geq$25 seconds of spike phenomena and δ and θ waves on the electroencephalogram). Pulse rate provides further evidence of a generalised seizure because it increases by 50–75% during a seizure and this increase persists for longer than the seizure. As mentioned above, prolactin secretion increases following a generalised seizure and measurements of prolactin approximately 30 minutes following ECT may be helpful if patients do not respond to apparently adequate seizures.

The 'dose' of electricity administered during ECT is referred to as the stimulus and is usually measured in units of electrical charge, millicoulombs (mC). The stimulus must be greater than the seizure threshold, the minimum stimulus capable of inducing a generalised seizure. The seizure threshold:

- may vary up to 40 fold between individuals within the range 25 to 800 mC and
- increases progressively by up to 200% during a course of ECT.

The factors known to increase the seizure threshold for ECT are listed in Box 17.1. The seizure threshold for ECT is reduced by caffeine, hyperventilation and hypoxia.

Box 17.1: Factors known to increase and reduce the seizure threshold for electroconvulsive therapy	
Fixed	Increasing age
	Male sex
	Baldness
	Thick skull (constitutional or Paget's disease)
	Bilateral electrode placement
	A course of electroconvulsive therapy
Modifiable	Antiepileptic, benzodiazepine and barbiturate drugs
	Dehydration
	Poor electrode contact with scalp

The stimulus administered at the initial ECT treatment may be either predetermined or calculated by dose titration. Predetermined ECT stimuli are listed in tables provided by the manufacturers of ECT treatment machines. They take account of age and sex and have been found by experience to effectively induce a seizure in 80% of treated individuals. Predetermined stimuli are easy to employ but a proportion of patients will receive stimuli significantly greater than their seizure threshold and this may increase cognitive adverse effects.

Dose titration involves administering a stimulus (50–75 mC) at the initial ECT treatment that will only induce a seizure in a minority of patients and then restimulating with progressively larger stimuli until a seizure occurs. This will be just above the seizure threshold and future administrations should be at 150% or 200% of this. This method is somewhat complex to employ and patients receive several stimuli at the initial ECT treatment. However, excessive stimulation is avoided thereafter and this may reduce cognitive adverse effects.

The seizure threshold increases progressively during a course of ECT and it may therefore be necessary to progressively increase the stimulus administered. Evidence of an increasing seizure threshold is provided by progressive reduction in the duration of the generalised seizure following subsequent administrations of ECT.

It is usual to administer ECT two or three times per week and an effective course of ECT may require from 8 to 20 treatments in the case of depression. Catatonia usually responds to fewer treatments while patients with mania may require more.

Maintenance electroconvulsive therapy

Maintenance ECT administered every 2 to 4 weeks was commonplace before the introduction of AD drugs but is now less frequently employed. However, depressed patients usually only receive ECT when AD drugs have proved ineffective. It therefore seems unreasonable to expect that AD drugs that have proven ineffective in treating depression will prove effective in preventing it recurring. It may be more reasonable to expect that ECT which has proven effective in treating depression will also prove effective in preventing it recurring. Research is lacking in this area but clinical experience confirms the efficacy and safety of maintenance ECT for a proportion of patients.

Safety

General adverse effects

ECT was initially administered to patients who were not anaesthetised and had not been treated with muscle relaxants. A mortality rate of 0.1% was recorded and a significant proportion of patients suffered vertebral compression fractures. The contemporary administration of ECT involves pre-oxygenation, anaesthesia, the administration of muscle relaxants and electrocardiographic and electroencephalographic monitoring. It is associated with a mortality rate of 0.002% and a morbidity rate of approximately 0.01%.

The most common adverse effects patients who receive ECT may experience are nausea, headache and myalgia. These quickly resolve with the passage of time or with symptomatic treatment. Cardiac arrhythmias are relatively common during treatment and immediately afterwards. These usually resolve without specific treatment.

The most serious adverse effects that may be experienced include prolonged seizures including status epilepticus, prolonged apnoea, laryngospasm and cardiac failure.

The risks associated with ECT are increased in patients who have:

- increased intracranial pressure
- cardiac failure caused by a recent myocardial infarction
- severe hypertension, particularly if associated with phaeochromocytoma
- an evolving cerebrovascular haemorrhage and
- retinal detachment.

It is important to note that there are no absolute contraindications to ECT. The above represent relative contraindications that must be weighed, along with the risk of anaesthesia, against the potential benefits of ECT for any individual patient.

Cognitive impairment

Almost all patients experience a period of confusion immediately following ECT. This is caused by the combined effects of anaesthesia and a generalised seizure and usually resolves without specific treatment and within a few hours.

Transient memory impairment is also experienced by almost all patients following ECT. This may be for either of or both events before ECT (retrograde amnesia) or subsequent to ECT (anterograde or post-traumatic amnesia). It usually resolves within weeks to months although it is not uncommon for patients to experience permanent loss of memory for some pre- and post-ECT events. Patients are rarely distressed by this memory impairment and recognise that it was caused by ECT and/or anaesthesia and that they are currently fully capable of learning and retaining new memories.

In contrast, some patients experience prolonged memory impairment following ECT and are understandably distressed by it. This memory impairment may involve not only prolonged retrograde and anterograde amnesia as described above but also persistent subjective difficulty in learning and retaining new memories. Prolonged memory impairment is more likely to develop following ECT involving a high frequency of treatments, a high absolute number of treatments, bilateral electrode placement, higher stimulus intensity and/or concomitant treatment with AD and other psychotropic drugs. The patho-physiology of prolonged memory impairment is poorly understood and may involve the effects of ECT itself or the interaction of ECT with the AD drugs that almost all patients receiving ECT are also taking. Memory impairment is also a feature of depression, schizophrenia and bipolar disorder, the diseases ECT is most often employed to treat.

It is often stated that there is no evidence that ECT causes brain damage. In fact it is more accurate to state that there is clear evidence that ECT does not cause brain damage. Thus structural neuroimaging studies reveal no changes following ECT and post-mortem studies do not differentiate neuropathologically between the brains of individuals who have been treated with ECT and those who have not.

Phototherapy

Phototherapy, first reported by Rosenthal et al (1984), is now a key treatment for winter depression.

Mechanism of action of phototherapy

It has long been known that circadian and seasonal rhythms in animals are controlled by variations in ambient light. These exert their effect via a system of neurones that extends from the retina via the supra-chiasmatic nucleus to the hypothalamus and thence to the endocrine system. Humans are subject to similar influences and winter depression may occur in individuals who are susceptible to a reduction in ambient light. Phototherapy is thought to reduce depressive symptoms by providing light 'replacement therapy' that modifies the hormones and biogenic amines that control mood. Neumeister et al (1998) have shown, for example, that both experimental tryptophan depletion and experimental catecholamine depletion (see Chapter 9) neutralise the beneficial effects of phototherapy.

Efficacy

Phototherapy is recommended for the treatment of winter depression, particularly in patients who eat and sleep excessively. It cannot be recommended for any other psychiatric disorder at this time but it is being investigated in sleep cycle disorders associated with shift work, intercontinental air travel and ageing. There is no NICE guidance currently available on phototherapy.

Phototherapy is administered via daily exposure for 30–60 minutes to light boxes positioned at eye level that contain fluorescent tubes and emit up to 10,000 lux. Less-powerful light boxes require periods of daily exposure of up to 2 hours. Light boxes do not emit ultraviolet light. Phototherapy may be administered in combination with AD drugs.

Phototherapy, if effective, should be continued until the hours of daylight increase and natural remission from winter depression is expected. Prophylactic phototherapy, initiated before the anticipated onset of winter depression, is effective in some patients.

Safety

Patients being treated with phototherapy may experience irritation of the eyes, headache and insomnia (which may be reduced by avoiding evening treatments).

There are no contraindications to phototherapy but induction of mania in depressed patients with unrecognised bipolar disorder is a theoretical risk.

Transcranial magnetic stimulation

In contrast to both ECT and phototherapy, TMS must currently be regarded as an experimental treatment for psychiatric disorders.

Magnetic stimulation of the brain has been used by neuro-physiologists for over a decade. For example movement in the right arm induced by magnetic stimulation of the left pre-frontal cortex confirms that the intervening neural systems are intact. TMS is now being investigated in the treatment of psychiatric disorders and in particular as a potential replacement for ECT. The attractiveness of a non-invasive, well-tolerated treatment will be apparent.

Mechanism of action of transcranial magnetic stimulation

TMS machines administer magnetic stimuli at up to 50 Hz via coils placed on the head. This induces electrical currents in the brain and these either increase or reduce brain activity for a short time.

Efficacy

TMS remains an experimental treatment. It has been investigated in obsessive compulsive disorder and a number of neurological disorders but it is in depression that most research is being undertaken. For example George et al (1997) reported that TMS at 20 Hz was superior to placebo TMS in reducing mean Hamilton depression scale scores in 12 depressed patients while a recent review concluded that published data support an antidepressant effect of high-frequency repetitive TMS administered to the left prefrontal cortex (Gershon et al, 2003).

Safety

TMS is non-invasive and appears to be free of significant adverse effects. Behavioural and neuropathological changes have not been noted in animals exposed to many thousands of TMS stimuli.

References and further reading

Cooney J (2005) Psychosurgery and ECT In: Core Psychiatry (Eds Wright P, Stern J, Phelan M) (2nd Edition). Edinburgh, Elsevier Saunders, pp. 611–619.

Freeman C (1995) The ECT Handbook (The Second Report of the Royal College of Psychiatrists Special Committee on ECT). London, Royal College of Psychiatrists, pp. 37–87.

George MS, Wassermann EM, Kimbrell TA et al (1997) Mood improvement following daily left prefrontal repetitive transcranial magnetic stimulation in patients with depression: a placebo-controlled crossover trial. American Journal of Psychiatry 154:1752–1756.

Gershon AA, Dannon PN, Grunhaus L (2003) Transcranial magnetic stimulation in the treatment of depression. American Journal of Psychiatry 160(5):835–845.

National Institute for Clinical Excellence – Guidance on the use of electroconvulsive therapy (Apr 2003) available online at http://www.nice.org.uk/pdf/59ectfullguidance.pdf (accessed July 2005).

Neumeister A et al (1998) Effects of tryptophan depletion versus catecholamine depletion in patients with seasonal affective disorder in remission with light therapy. Archives of General Psychiatry 55:524–530.

Rosenthal NE, Sack DA, Gillin JC et al (1984) Seasonal affective disorder. A description of the syndrome and preliminary findings with light therapy. Archives of General Psychiatry 41(1):72–80.

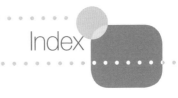

C